A PERSONAL WELLNESS PROGRAM

Stick With EXERCISE

For A Lifetime

HOW TO ENJOY EVERY MINUTE OF IT!

ROBERT HOPPER, PhD

CreateSpace

Library of Congress cataloging-in-publication data is available from the Library of Congress.

10 9 8 7 6 5 4 3

ISBN 1-467-90993-9

Design by MICHAEL BESSIRE

Manufactured in the United States of America

FIRST EDITION: JULY 2012

This book is dedicated to the 7 out of 10 Americans who have tried and failed with exercise—but have yet to give up on achieving an active lifestyle.

Contents

Forewords

Taking that First Step

Early on in life I discovered the power of goal-setting. At age 7, I joined a swim club; I had a clear objective in mind. My mother had signed me up for ballet—I figured if I agreed to join the swim club, I could get out of dance classes. Score!

Initially I saw swimming as splashy workouts and playtime with friends. As I progressed, it became more about competition. At 14, I set my first national age-group records. I liked swimming, but it was the feeling of success and accomplishment that made me love it. At 15, I made the Olympic team and Jim Montrella, my coach, created a totally focused workout for me. As coach and athlete, Jim and I evolved together. We experienced the full spectrum of frustrations and elations. At times Jim put the fear of God in me—but he kept me motivated. It was Jim who made me believe I could do these things I never thought I could do.

Years later, I became a swimming coach myself. At first I was frustrated that my students didn't have the same motivation as I did at their age. I had to learn how to accept a different level of performance, but I came to love the satisfaction that arose from motivating students and fostering their sense of accomplishment.

The world of sports and the role of physical activity in my life have continued to change over time. Today I look at exercise in terms of the social aspects and personal health. I never swim. As what Dr. Robert Hopper calls an "everyday athlete," I work out at home and I like to walk with friends. Staying active makes me feel good. Walking keeps me moving, and it has a relaxed camaraderie that's supportive and encouraging.

In his insightful book, Dr. Hopper points out that friends, neighbors, family members, classmates, and teachers are all great sources of support for "everyday athletes." Another invaluable theme of this book: exercise should be fun. And Dr. Hopper encourages everyone keen to develop an exercise habit to picture any physical activity they've ever dreamed of doing, then take that first step...and try doing it! For anyone of any ability seeking an active lifestyle, *Stick with Exercise for a Lifetime* is a book to read and reread. It will inspire you to make a leap of faith—and to keep making those leaps. If your sport speaks to you, you can and will find the time.

The sport I used to daydream about is stand-up paddling. I probably thought about doing it for two years. One day I went for a walk and ran into my neighbor, Jericho Poppler [the champion surfer and longboarder]. She knew I'd wanted to try stand-up paddling for ages so she bugged me about it. She said, "You can do it! It'll be fun!"

Now I want to get my own board. I wasn't all that great at balancing the first time, but I really liked the serenity of it—and being on the water instead of in it.

–**Susie Atwood,** *two-time Olympic Medalist*
Held 24 American and World Records
Held 23 National Championship Swimming Titles
Member, International Swimming Hall of Fame

Embracing the Shift from Goal to Process

As a kid, I was lucky I always had good coaches, good mentors, and good teachers. My swimming and water polo coaches had great patience with me and they were excellent motivators. I started my own coaching career at 19—and once again I was lucky. Among my first students was a 7-year-old swimmer named Susie Atwood who went on to become an Olympic champion.

Like all super-athletes, Susie possessed not just extraordinary physical talent but also an exceptional intellect, a well-developed sense of self, and a keen ability to assimilate processes from an early age. She also had wonderful support and encouragement from her family and teammates. By age 8, Susie had set her first national record. Susie liked swimming and she loved winning. At the time, I saw it as my job to keep her winning—so I pushed her hard to improve.

Athletic competition always offers the opportunity for self-improvement. A good coach finds ways for that improvement to be pleasurable and meaningful. What I learned from Susie was that at times I needed to ease up on my own goals about winning in order to make her workouts and training more enjoyable. To best develop her talent, I needed to develop more patience. This shift in outlook from goal to process proved to be an invaluable career and life lesson.

I see coaches today who are the same as I was when I started out—overly results-oriented and pushing too hard. And I see too many Americans in general falling into this same trap with exercise—which is why I'm so excited about this book. It has the potential to help so many people succeed with exercise. An exercise program is not about winning; it's not a short-term problem to fix with a grueling stint at the gym. It's a lifelong process that should bring satisfaction and pleasure.

In *Stick with Exercise for a Lifetime*, my respected colleague and friend Dr. Robert Hopper delivers this refreshingly simple and long overdue message in multiple contexts that show you exactly how to embrace that process, how to get support for your efforts, and how to integrate exercise into a daily routine.

Dr. Hopper's point is to take your time—find a physical activity you truly enjoy and be the champion of yourself! Getting that message—gently making that mental shift—gives us all so many opportunities to find our way to a happier, healthier way of life.

> **–Jim Montrella,** *Olympic coach*
> *Member, American Swimming Coaches Hall of Fame*

Section One

Chapter I

FUN

The solution for your best-laid plans

One morning as I was working on a draft of this book at my neighborhood Starbucks, a woman at a nearby table turned to me and said, "You look so intent. What are you working on?" I told her I was writing a book on how to stick with an exercise program for a lifetime. Her response was strong and immediate. "Let me know when you complete the book," she said. "I want a copy!"

> "The more pleasure you get from physical activity, the more likely it is you'll want to engage in more of it."

That same response occurs nearly every time I mention this topic. So many people I meet are frustrated with making New Year's resolutions to exercise regularly, only to fail after a matter of months or weeks. Sometimes even days.

Every year, millions of Americans begin an exercise program to lose weight for the summer, to get ready for a class reunion, to somehow transform their lifestyle to improve their health and fitness. Somehow, they never reach those goals. While visions of improved health and fitness—not to mention looking and feeling great—can get most of us started on an exercise program, they're notoriously weak motivators over the long haul.

The purpose of this book is to teach you how to succeed with exercise for that long haul; to share the secrets of top athletes on what makes it possible—even easy—to stick with exercise for a lifetime. Whether it's Wimbledon Champion tennis player Serena Williams, Olympic swimmer Michael Phelps, or golf legend Tiger Woods, top athletes have relied on a set of best practices at the start of their careers that help them get to the highest levels of their sport.

In the following chapters, you'll learn about the best practices for exercise success that will help you achieve your goals. You'll also learn about Championship Moments and the key mental techniques to help you "just do it"—to overcome the impulse to drop out of your fitness program. With these tools, you'll have the power to overcome the obstacles that stand between you and your healthiest, most vibrant self. Best of all, you'll have fun doing it!

During my years as a college swimming coach and assistant professor in physical education, and later, when I developed corporate wellness programs, I noticed that most people I worked with already knew about the health benefits of regular physical activity. They understood that regular exercise was a key part of any weight loss and maintenance program, that brisk exercise was a good way to relieve stress, and that vigorous physical activity was beneficial to the heart and circulatory system.

Their problem was that they just couldn't seem to stay with a program for very long. This perplexed me. All my life, exercise came naturally. An only child, I was fortunate to have active role models. My mom was a competitive swimmer through her 20s and 30s; she won a national championship and almost made it to the Olympics. She taught me to swim and encouraged me to have fun in our little backyard pool. I also had fun on the playground. In elementary school, I was the king of recess. Whether it was softball, basketball, or punch ball, I loved games and physical activities. My dad loved tennis, and I tagged along and soon started playing sets with my friends. I naively grew up thinking exercise should be instinctive and effortless for everyone. Research for this book taught me otherwise.

If you've failed or had limited success with exercise programs in the past, you are not alone. A recent Centers for Disease Control and Prevention national health survey showed that just three in ten adults in the United States get adequate exercise; another three in ten get a little exercise, and a substantial four in ten don't exercise at all. That's right—that means 70 percent of adults don't get adequate exercise.[1]

Why would so many people have difficulty sticking with something as essential as exercise when it has such obvious benefits? Regular physical activity plays a role in reducing risk for heart disease, cancer, diabetes, and stroke. It helps people maintain a healthy weight and manage stress. This sad state of affairs certainly can't be blamed on a lack of available information on the subject.

Tens of thousands of articles and books have been written about exercise, starting with physician Kenneth H. Cooper's revolutionary book *Aerobics* in 1968. This book launched the fitness revolution of the 1970s.[2] Suddenly, people were jogging in place on every street corner, holding a hand against a wrist or throat, monitoring their heart rates. Today, you can read endlessly about which exercises to do, how often to do them, how vigorously to do them, what kind of equipment to use for your routine, how to capture and track your biometric data on phones and laptops, what to wear to the gym....

Curiously absent from all this discourse is the topic of how to stick with an exercise program.

Choose your path to success

Imagine yourself in climbing gear, standing at the base of towering "Mount Fitness." In front of you are two signs. The one labeled "Traditional" points to a well-paved route that scales a moderately steep slope and lands you at the breathtaking summit. The other sign, labeled "Alternate," directs you to a meandering trail bordered by wildflowers. The trail traverses the face of the mountain, with each loop ascending a little higher, until it eventually reaches that same breathtaking summit.

Which route will you take? The routes represent two very different approaches to exercise, health, and fitness. The traditional route usually involves signing up at a gym and counting your way down to a buff physique: doing reps, sweating on the treadmill. By dedicating yourself to a rigorous traditional fitness center program, you'll be vibrantly healthy and fit—as long as you keep up the routine.

But if you've tried gym workouts and don't like them—or, try as you might, you just can't seem to stick with them—there's the other choice.

On the alternate route, you choose from a wide range of physical activities, basing your choices on the level of fun, enjoyment, and satisfaction each provides. Your alternate route exercise program might include activities like bowling, bocce, kayaking, yoga, scuba diving, or salsa dancing. You pursue a physical activity program with the goal of having fun, learning new skills, and improving performance. That's right: health and fitness are not the overt goals of this program, but they're natural *byproducts*—the side benefits of having fun with regular physical activity. In other words, the goal is to develop your talent in one or more physical activities that you enjoy.

At the core of this alternate approach is the idea that genuinely enjoying an activity, learning new skills, improving performance, and developing talent serve as powerful motivators to stick with exercise. This book is a guide to taking that approach.

Let's take a quick look at the traditional route and then contrast that with an example of the alternate route.

The traditional route

Consider Joan, whose physical fitness program entails exercising three to four times a week at a nearby gym. An exercise professional designed Joan's program, basing it on fitness guidelines of the American College of

Sports Medicine and the American Heart Association, which we'll discuss in further detail in Chapter Five. Over several years, Joan develops cardiovascular endurance, muscular strength, and good flexibility. Regular exercise helps her achieve her ideal weight, look and feel younger, and decrease her risk of heart disease, cancer, diabetes, and stroke. For Joan and millions of Americans like her, this traditional approach to exercise has been a resounding success. For many more Americans, however, this approach has failed.

The alternate route

The alternate route is about pursuing a physical activity program with the goal of having fun. It's the active lifestyle approach. While health and fitness are not the explicit goals of such a program, they're the natural side benefits of having fun while engaging in pleasurable physical activities.

Bill and Sue choose this alternate approach, opting to develop their talent in swing dance. One evening they happen by their local recreation center and see people inside taking a swing dancing class. It looks like fun. While they've never been especially good dancers, they figure they can do as well as the students inside. What the heck—maybe they'll enjoy learning the basic dance steps. As novices, they enroll in a beginning class and wind up taking the course twice, partly because they want to master the basic steps but mostly because it's a blast.

Over the next few years, Bill and Sue complete all the beginning and intermediate series classes and start in on their advanced skills. They feel a sense of satisfaction as they improve, dancing three or four times a week in classes or at area clubs. They both look and feel more vibrant. They even enter a local dance competition. While they focus on having fun, learning new skills, and improving performance, their health and fitness improve almost effortlessly.

Bill and Sue could substitute other activities with the same results. For instance, they could try classes in country, folk, belly, ballroom, Polynesian, or another style of dance. Or, they could select from a bounty of other leisure activities like ice-skating, waterskiing, martial arts, rollerblading, outrigger canoeing, yoga, and more. With regular lessons, they'll progress through the beginning, intermediate, and advanced classes. Their net gain will be the satisfaction that comes from talent development—as well as improved health and fitness, the side benefits that arise from having fun with regular exercise.

Because talent development is going to play a vital role in your exercise program, let's look at some time-tested, proven strategies you can use to reach your potential. For many of us, the key to exercise success lies in the mental shift from improving health and fitness to the goal of developing your talent in one or more physical activities.

A look at peak performers

The business world concept of "best practices" may offer a solution to the millions of Americans who lack adequate exercise. Forward-thinking companies identify the best practices of highly successful, peak-performing personnel, and teach those practices to their other employees with the goal of increasing productivity and profits. What would happen if we applied that best practices model to the challenge of sticking with exercise?

Well, who comes to mind when you think of the most successful, peak performing exercisers in the country? Certainly professional athletes belong to that group. While your mind may jump to the pros you see on TV, how about the millions of kids across America who participate in youth sports and age-group competitions. Consider high school teens who take part in after-school sports, as well as college students participating in intramural sports and those who dedicate two to four hours each day to National Collegiate Athletic Association teams.

Add to that growing group of peak performers those adults who participate in organized sports and active leisure pursuits. Your coworkers who walk, run, or ride in charity events are athletes. That friend hooked on Pilates or aerobic dance is an athlete. The neighbors who play tennis every weekend—they're athletes, too. So are regular hikers, belly dancers, bowlers, mountain bikers, trail runners, snowboarders, surfers, skydivers, and active participants in recreational softball, lacrosse, ping-pong, and beach volleyball. Your buddy who practices yoga is an athlete, and so is your sister-in-law who spends every afternoon digging, hoeing, and planting in the garden.

All of these people—young and old, beginners or advanced devotees—are among the most successful exercisers in America. They're what I call "everyday athletes," people who include exercise instinctively as part of their daily routine. Do they know something you don't know? Do they have a set of best practices that can help them succeed? Are these everyday athletes inadvertently using the same set of best practices used by world-class pros? Could it be that your strategy for success will be to use these tools to increase the pleasure you get from participating in physical activities?

The answer is a resounding yes!

A best practices approach

As a kid, I loved swimming. I never had problems sticking with physical activities. As a young adult, things changed. I had difficulty building my exercise program around activities such as jogging, stationary cycling, and weight training. I strived to adhere to standard fitness guidelines, but I wasn't especially successful. Later, the problem became obvious: I didn't enjoy fitness activities. On the other hand, I was blissfully successful in leisure and recreational activities like tennis, golf, skiing, swimming, surfing, scuba diving, and dancing. It was these activities that sustained my good health and fitness.

Examining my athletic experiences, I identified several key factors, or best practices, that were vital to my success. I unconsciously relied on certain strategies that made it easier to stick with exercise. What were they?

My first thought was that swimming was fun. As far as I could tell, every other kid involved in sports and games was having a great time. Could it be that fun was a key ingredient? It seems only logical that the odds of succeeding with exercise over a lifetime would be greatly increased if you were having the time of your life while pursuing it.

I kept adding to my list of best practices. All athletes have a coach to teach them skills, provide motivation, and guide their careers. And they all belong to a team. Could it be that the effects of having a coach and belonging to a team are more keys to long-term exercise success?

I also knew that time was rarely a problem for athletes—because practice times are etched in granite. Every young athlete begins practice right after school. Did athletes practice time management skills that were vital for success? And what about goals? For myself and other swimmers, we always set our goals a little higher each season. Pursuing these goals was fun, and when we reached them we enjoyed rewards. Obvious rewards were ribbons, medals, trophies, and mentions in the school and local papers. More important though, were the rewards of respect and recognition from our teachers and peers.

I remember when I got my All-America award in high school and put the patch on my letterman's jacket. Suddenly girls who never noticed me began to show a little interest! I also remember the pride I felt. In addition, athletes at all levels engage in a supplementary fitness program—in some form of strength or cardio training—to improve their performance. Could this desire to improve performance provide the additional motivation needed to succeed with a fitness program?

Finally, over time athletes learn how to get themselves to do the hard work required to succeed. They develop mental techniques that enable them to "just do it"—to stick with their plans and goals. Could learning such techniques—mastering what I call Championship Moments—help the average person succeed with exercise long term?

My findings suggested that what once helped me succeed with swimming—indeed, what helps world-class athletes develop their talent—was a fairly universal set of practices with something in common: they begin and end with pleasure.

I went on to discover that a monumental body of research on human talent development backs up this conclusion. Groundbreaking studies undertaken by educational psychologist Benjamin S. Bloom at the University of Chicago through the 1980s led to the establishment of a whole new field of research in talent development.[3] Moreover, the U.S. Olympic Committee referenced Bloom's findings in its own studies on the development of Olympic athletes.[4]

Reading further, I was excited to find that the best practices I relied upon are indeed used by world-class swimmers, tennis players, gymnasts, ping-pong players, marathon runners, and athletes of every stripe. In addition, these best practices span multiple disciplines, playing a key role in talent development not only in sports but also in everything from mathematics to music.

In this book, we'll explore each of these practices—the best practices for exercise success—in detail. Note that all of them contribute to the pleasure that comes from learning new skills and improving performance.

1	*Have fun*
2	*Work with a coach*
3	*Join a team*
4	*Schedule time for play and practice*
5	*Enhance performance with a supplementary fitness program*
6	*Set goals for continuous improvement*
7	*Make winning choices at Championship Moments*

The secret to long-term success with exercise involves using these best practices to maximize your enjoyment of any physical activity. In upcoming chapters, you'll learn more about how athletes draw on these practices and how you can easily apply a similar approach to your own exercise program. But first, it's time to make some of the most important choices in your life. On the next few pages, you'll find a checklist of potential lifetime activities that millions of Americans of all ages enjoy on a regular basis.

Your challenge—and it's an easy one—is to identify the activities you think would be genuinely fun to do over a lifetime. It's human nature that you'll like some choices more than others. What matters is that finding even *one* activity you enjoy year-round can provide a lifetime of enjoyment, fitness, and health.

Lifetime sports

In considering all the sports to choose from, don't expect to find your activity for life right off the bat. Kids often try a number of different sports before they find the one they like the most. Expect the same for yourself. There's an element of chance in the selection of your lifetime activity. Much like finding a mate, the only way to know what's right for you is to try a 'dating' period. You may choose one activity and later decide it wasn't quite what you thought. Or you may try a variety of activities, and the one you thought you'd enjoy the least might end up being your favorite.

In this book, I don't recommend any specific physical activities. I only recommend you choose activities that you think will be enjoyable, satisfying, and, above all, fun. For one person, lifting weights or working out on an elliptical machine will be thrilling; for another, it will be pure boredom.

The choice is yours

Put a check mark (✔) in front of all the activities you think might be fun to learn. If you have doubts about your ability to learn new skills—or about being in good enough physical condition to participate—put those doubts aside for now and we'll address them later. For now, consider the following:

➤ *Assume you have the physical fitness required to join in any activity you choose.*

➤ *Assume you can easily learn the skills to enjoy that activity. For the time it takes you to complete your checklist, focus exclusively on finding activities that stir your soul.*

➤ *Be daring! Embrace your wildest fantasies! If you've dreamed about snorkeling or scuba diving a coral reef off Hawaii or the Bahamas, be sure to put a check mark (✔) by snorkeling and/or scuba diving—even if you can't swim.*

➤ *For activities on your list that strike you as especially exciting, add a heart (♥) next to the check mark. Your list should be all about activities that stir your soul.*

If you can find activities that ignite a passion, you virtually guarantee success, no matter who tells you it's impossible.

YOUR LIFETIME SPORTS

TRADITIONAL ROUTE ACTIVITIES

___ Aerobic exercise, circuit training, elliptical trainer, resistance training, rowing machine, spinning/stationary bike, treadmill, weight training, etc.

ALTERNATE ROUTE ACTIVITIES

___ Aerobic dance

___ Aqua aerobics, water aerobics

___ Archery

___ Backpacking

___ Badminton

___ Ballet

___ Ballroom dance

___ Basketball

___ Belly dancing

___ Bicycle riding

___ Bocce, pétanque

___ Bodysurfing

___ Boogie boarding

___ Bowling

___ Boxing

___ Bungee jumping

___ Camping

___ Canoeing

___ Climbing, mountaineering

___ Country-western dance

___ Cricket

___ Croquet

___ Curling

___ Dirt bike riding

___ Fencing

___ Football

___ Folk dancing

___ Free diving

___ Frisbee, ultimate Frisbee

___ Frisbee golf

___ Gardening

___ Golf

___ Gymnastics

___ Handball

___ Hiking

___ Hip-hop dance

___ Horseback riding

___ Hula, Polynesian dance

___ Ice climbing

___ Ice dancing

___ Ice hockey

___ Ice-skating

___ Jai alai

___ Jet-skiing

___ Kayaking

___ Kickboxing

___ Kiteboarding

___ Lacrosse

___ Latin dance

___ Lawn bowling

___ Marathons

___ Martial arts, judo, karate

___ Mountain biking

___ Modern, jazz dance

___ Paddling, outrigger
canoeing

___ Paragliding

___ Parkour

___ Pilates

___ Ping-pong

___ Polo

___ Racquetball

___ River rafting, white-water
rafting

___ Rock climbing

___ Roller-skating

___ Rollerblading,
in-line skating

___ Rowing, sculling

___ Rugby

___ Running, jogging,
trail running

___ Sailing

___ Salsa dance

___ Scuba diving

___ Skateboarding

___ Skiing, cross-country
or downhill

___ Skydiving

___ Snorkeling

___ Snowboarding

___ Snowmobiling

___ Snowshoeing

___ Soccer

___ Softball

___ Square dance

___ Squash

___ Stand-up paddling

___ Stretching

___ Surfing

___ Swimming

___ Swing dance

___ Tae Bo

___ Tai chi

___ Tap dance

___ Tennis

___ Triathlons

___ Track

___ Volleyball

___ Walking

___ Water polo

___ Waterskiing

___ Windsurfing

___ Yoga

___ Zip-lining

___ Zumba

___ Other: _____

Take a second look

Let me be perfectly clear: if you can't swim, but think swimming would be fun, by all means check off swimming. Remember, at one time neither world-champion surfer Kelly Slater nor Olympic medalist Michael Phelps even knew how to tread water. I've taught hundreds of adults how to swim; from an instructor's perspective, it's easy to take nonswimmers and turn them into swimmers. And if you think skydiving, boogie boarding, snorkeling, soccer, polo, or ballet would be fun—but have never skydived, boogie boarded, snorkeled, kicked a soccer ball, mounted a horse, or done a plié—check them off. It's easy to learn physical activities, as you'll find in the next chapter.

Now take a second look at the list of lifetime sports. Did you check off all the activities you *really* thought might be fun? Or did you skip an activity such as, say, fencing, football, stand-up paddling, or modern dance because you thought it might be too hard to learn? Perhaps you left out martial arts since you've never done it before.

If you left out *any* activities that your gut tells you could be fun, go back and put a check mark by those activities.

On the other hand, did you include some activities because they're simple and convenient, but in truth you don't think they'd be fun? Did you choose a fitness activity like jogging simply because there's a park nearby—but you feel jogging would boring? If you weren't completely honest with yourself—if you chose activities that didn't strike you as all that much fun—go back and erase those check marks. The end result should be a list of activities you think would undoubtedly be fun to learn.

By now, a question may be creeping into your mind: since some of these activities are not nearly as vigorous as traditional fitness activities, will the less vigorous activities still improve your health and fitness? The answer is yes!

Keep in mind that your primary goal is to be physically active on a regular basis for a lifetime. When you're having fun being physically active, health and fitness are the side benefits.

Of course, if you choose more vigorous lifetime sports, you'll develop a greater amount of physical fitness as you improve. But there's more to that story. There's a paradox about exercise that validates most any physical activity.

The paradox of fun

The more pleasure you derive from an activity—as measured by fun, enjoyment, and satisfaction—the more likely it is you'll want to engage in more vigorous physical fitness activities to improve your performance. Remember, all athletes rely on a supplementary fitness program to improve their performance.

If you focus initially on fun, that can happen to you as well. You may take up dancing, tennis, or snowboarding—but as you develop your talent in your lifetime sport, you may want to enroll in an aerobics class, a stretching class, or lift a few weights in order to be stronger and perform better at that sport.

THE NEXT STEP

Before we go further, try to make a quick decision: if you checked off more than one activity you thought would be fun, decide which one you want to learn first. It will enhance your learning as you read upcoming chapters if you can immediately relate them to a particular activity.

In the next chapter, you'll discover how to easily learn the skills of something you've never done before.

Chapter Two

COACH

The guide to reaching your milestones

Every world-class athlete has a coach—often a series of coaches—and rarely achieves excellence without one. The most important of these coaches is the first one, perhaps a parent but more likely a beginning-level instructor good at working with kids. If that first coach fails at making a sport fun, the young pro-athlete-to-be might quit right at the start.

In this chapter, you will learn how a beginning-level coach can transform you into someone who knows the basic skills of your chosen physical activity and enjoys doing it on a regular basis.

▶▶

"Remember, at one time, Olympic swimmer Dara Torres didn't know the freestyle."

Remember, at one time Olympic swimmer Dara Torres didn't know the freestyle, Wimbledon tennis legend Serena Williams had never held a racket, and world champion surfer Kelly Slater had yet to catch a wave. All of them started out at the same place you may be now—never having done the activity before—and they all started with lessons.

Your initial coach may be a folk dancing or riding teacher, a water aerobics class leader, maybe a personal trainer or a paragliding instructor. These teachers, instructors, or class leaders can help you succeed where you might have failed in the past. Specifically, they can help you through those first steps toward achieving long-term success with exercise.

What we can learn from athletes

Even skiers like Lindsey Vonn, the U.S. downhill gold medalist at the 2010 Vancouver Winter Olympics, had to learn the basic steps when first introduced to their future sport. Vonn's father, a onetime national junior champion, had his daughter on skis at age 3.[5] But why do those children who grow up to become world-class athletes stay involved in a sport after that initial introduction? Their coaches help them through three critical steps.

TED LEARNS THE SNOWPLOW *Ted inhales the crisp winter air. He has never skied. Now, at age 44, he and his fellow students face their first hills. Their instructor has showed the class of six how to put on skis and get comfortable standing, how to traverse a gentle slope and make a snowplow turn, how to control speed, and how to stop. Before the lesson, Ted felt intimidated by the sport, but the instructor's encouragement and systematic progression has made it easy for him to learn each new skill. By the end of the lesson, he's zipping down the gentle hill, beaming proudly at friends watching the action from the lodge.*

Like any new skier who goes on to be successful at the sport, Ted goes through a progression: his first step is a good initial experience; the second step is early success; and the third, and perhaps most vital step, is continuous improvement. Let's look at how coaches help kids navigate these steps and how a coach can help you do the same.

THE ABC'S OF LONG-TERM SUCCESS

A good initial experience

Picture yourself as a child taking your first swimming lesson; if you have a good initial experience in the water, you look forward to your second lesson. Or imagine you've learned how to swim, and you've just joined a novice swim team. On the very first day, the coach has you in the water doing relays and playing games. While it seems like an hour of fun with your friends, those relays and games have you practicing the initial skills of competitive swimming. At dinner, bursting with enthusiasm, you tell your family how much you enjoyed the team.

After that experience, you certainly want to come back the next day. It's an hour of fun with your friends.

Kids usually start an activity because they think it will be fun. If their initial experience is less than positive, they'll probably quit and move on to something else. But if they enjoy it right from the start, they'll want to continue. This principle holds true with any age group. Remember Ted, who had never skied before? With the guidance of a good coach, he tackled the slopes and, by day's end, was elated by the experience.

A "coach"—also known as a teacher, trainer, instructor, or class leader—begins the process of creating a good initial experience by reserving the practice location, providing beginning-level equipment, and ensuring that the process of learning initial skills is enjoyable. Swimming teachers, for instance, know that if they create an enjoyable learning experience where the child has fun, learns to feel comfortable in the water, and, at the end of the lesson can perform a new skill, that child will want to return.

Early success

The second factor in whether a child will continue with a given sport is early success. Talent development studies have shown that all world-class athletes report early success—often within the first few months.[6] Doing well in the early stages creates a desire to continue. This occurs in virtually all endeavors of life. Early success creates the desire for *more success*.

A coach can take you step-by-step from being a non-participant to someone who knows the basic skills and enjoys participation. Somewhere along the way, you'll feel you've reached a new and improved default comfort level with physical activity. You'll be doing the beginning skills and having fun—and it will feel good.

Continuous improvement

An early victory launched my swimming career. I was 10. My first summer novice swim team ended with an evening meet wherein I won my first race—the 50-yard freestyle. I can still feel the exhilaration. My parents recognized my excitement, too, and enrolled me in a team that practiced year-round.

One of my first goals as a young swimmer was to break 30 seconds for the 50-yard freestyle—two laps up and back in a 25-yard pool. When I broke through the 30-second barrier at 29.5 seconds, I was really excited—and almost immediately had a new goal to break 29 seconds. Later that goal became 28 seconds, then 27....

It was fun chasing after these goals, but I couldn't have done it without a coach. If you watch an age-group team practice, you'll see a coach pull one swimmer aside, work with that swimmer for a few moments to make a correction, then send the swimmer back to practice laps. It's that regular instruction and coaching that helps young athletes quickly master new skills and improve their performance.

For you, taking lessons is the quickest and surest way to learn new skills and continually improve performance. As part of your plan for exercise success, make sure your lessons will be ongoing and that an instructor, teacher, or coach will play a continuing role in your development. Your coach's long-term plan should be to build on those early skills and guide you through the intermediate and advanced skills so you can experience many future successes.

Remember, your future teacher, instructor, class leader, or coach has already helped hundreds of students achieve the three milestones—a good initial experience, early success, and continuous improvement—and they can do the same for you.

PAM BLOWS UNDERWATER BUBBLES *At age 45, Pam decides to realize a long-held dream to scuba dive Hawaii's sparkling reefs. The main obstacle to that dream? Pam first needs to learn how to swim. One day she takes the plunge. She sets about researching who can teach her. The process turns out to be simple. Pam looks up area swimming pools and inquires about lessons. She visits facilities and clubs that offer lessons at convenient times. She joins the YMCA because it's close to home, suits her budget, and has beginning classes for adults. She also likes that the Y has a hot tub where she can warm up before class.*

Pam enrolls in a ten-session class, held on Saturday mornings. The class has five members, so the instructor can provide plenty of personal attention. The instructor's games make learning new skills fun. To start, the instructor has the group stand in the water, then submerge their faces to blow bubbles underwater and watch each other blow bubbles. Pam soon feels comfortable opening her eyes underwater. By her tenth lesson, she can swim comfortably across the pool.

Thanks to the guidance of a skilled coach, Pam has a good initial experience and early success. She continues improving with intermediate and advanced swimming lessons. When she can swim a mile, she takes scuba lessons. She heads to Hawaii to complete her scuba certification and fulfill her dream.

WHAT TO LOOK FOR IN A COACH

When the parents of most world-class athletes enroll their kids in lessons, talent development studies have shown that two simple factors tend to determine their choice of initial coach or instructor.[7] One factor benefits the child, the other benefits the parent. You'll want to consider these two factors in developing your new exercise program. Let's see how they affect you.

Skill with beginners

Parents of young athletes often look for instructors who have a good reputation for working with beginners. First and foremost, they want their kids to have a good first impression of the sport and have fun right from the start. You can do the same.

Find a coach who has a reputation for working well with beginners. You'll want an instructor who likes working with people who have no clue how to do an activity; who can transform those people into enthusiastic participants in a matter of weeks. This kind of coach no doubt gets a great deal of satisfaction from helping students get started.

Generally, a beginning series of lessons for golf, racquet sports, or dance ranges from six to ten lessons, often once a week. Starting from lesson one, the instructor will work hard to create an enjoyable initial experience, focusing on teaching the skills that foster early success.

Convenience

Parents today often function as chauffeurs for their kids, driving them to soccer practice, music lessons, and other after-school activities. Taking their child to activities located nearby is a big plus. Parents of top-performing young athletes are no different. Studies show that convenience is essential to the choice of beginning teacher.[8]

Early on, parents of top performers have no indication that their child has talent and will grow up to reach international levels of competition. Their primary interest is simply to expose their child to healthy activities.

In the beginning, convenience is paramount. Once such children show talent, however, their parents are willing to drive long distances to make sure they have good coaching.

Your choice of a coach should hinge on convenience as well. In today's world, where many people cite lack of time as a major constraint to regular exercise, finding an easily accessible instructor can be a critical step toward early success. Look for an instructor close to your home, or maybe on the route between home and your office if you plan to exercise right after work.

OTHER FACTORS

Group or private lessons

Beginning-level coaches like group lessons because they can reach a large number of people in the same hour-long lesson. Group lessons also provide an enjoyable way to start a new sport. The major benefits of group lessons? You get to learn with other like-minded beginners, and the cost of instruction is shared by the class members. On the downside, if there are six people in your class, you get one-sixth of your instructor's time for personal attention.

Private lessons—essentially one-on-one coaching—are also an excellent way to have an enjoyable initial experience and early success. While private lessons are more expensive, you get the instructor's full attention throughout the lesson, during both the instructional and practice phases. Having an instructor provide feedback while you're practicing a skill will accelerate learning a new sport.

You may want to try both types of lessons. Let's say you feel a bit anxious or reluctant about taking a class. Often, the person who teaches the beginners class may also teach individual lessons. Consider taking an initial private lesson, or maybe two to three, to see if you like the activity. This early handholding may be just the ticket to help you overcome your fears and help you feel comfortable joining a group class in the future.

Coach as personal guide

Your first coach will become your guide through the early stages of development in your sport. Even before you start your first lesson, the coach will tell you what to expect in the initial lessons. As you improve, he or she will lead you through subsequent steps, over time guiding you through the transformation from novice to confident, skilled participant.

This coach may take you through several series of lessons. Generally, you start with a beginning series of six to ten lessons. If you like that introductory class, your coach may encourage you to enroll in an advanced beginning class, followed by several intermediate-level classes and, eventually, the advanced classes that can keep you learning and developing your talent in your sport for many years to come. As your guide, the coach will tell you when it might be advisable to repeat a class.

Research shows that, in general, "mastery learning"—mastering skills at each level before you move forward—is the best way to learn a sport. Your coach will help you progress, and tell you when you're ready for the intermediate and advanced skills. Your coach may also provide the equipment you'll need in the beginning, or point you to the most cost-effective beginning-level equipment (both used and new), as well as when and how to best upgrade that equipment as you progress. Over all, your first coach can and should be a source of answers for all your questions about your new activity.

Note that I emphasize the idea of ongoing lessons because adults often take beginning-level lessons and then forge ahead on their own without further lessons or coaching. Here's the key point: if athletes at the pinnacle of success still rely on coaching to help them improve, assume you can benefit by doing the same.

Be coachable

Most coaches have chosen their field because they love the sport and enjoy helping students learn skills and become successful. You can make the process go more smoothly and quickly by being coachable.

Initiate the process by asking sincere questions, then taking action to make improvements. When I was a coach and an athlete came to me for help, it made my day. And when that athlete improved, I felt great. The biggest compliment a coach can receive is to see that you took a lesson to heart, practiced new skills, and showed obvious progress at the next lesson. Coaches love to work with people who want to improve. If you develop this kind of relationship, with trust in your coach's expertise and ability, you'll jet-propel your progress. Here are a few more tips for getting the most from coaching:

- *When your instructor walks from participant to participant—and you're next—be ready with any questions you might have.*
- *Be receptive to comments about what you may be doing wrong. When an instructor points out something that needs correcting and you do so, you will improve.*
- *When the instructor leaves, try to work right away on any skills you asked about. The instructor may glance back over a shoulder to see if you're taking the advice to heart. If you are, he or she will be encouraged to provide more feedback at future lessons.*
- *Practice between lessons. Instructors notice when you've practiced by your rate of improvement. If you advance because of their coaching, that encourages them to provide more feedback in the future—which in turn allows you to develop your talent that much faster!*
- *At the end of each class, thank the instructor for the lesson.*

In general, coachable people's actions show that they really want to learn—that they're willing to apply their instructor's suggestions.

HOW TO APPLY WHAT YOU'VE LEARNED

Where to find your first coach

Start with friends. One of the best ways to learn about a new lifetime sport is to talk to friends involved in a similar activity. If you have friends who do stretching classes, step aerobics, triathlons, enjoy the Texas two-step, play polo, water ski, or practice karate, they'll know where to find lessons in those sports, and may be able to recommend instructors who are good with beginners. They may even introduce you to the coach of their class, group, or club.

Recreation departments

City recreation departments often host beginning swimming and tennis lessons, all kinds of dance classes, and a variety of other indoor and outdoor activities. Go to your recreation department and pick up their class schedule, or look it up online. Then go to a session. Watch the instructor and participants in action. If the class seems fun and the instructor seems effective, sign up for the class.

Fitness centers, YMCAs, athletic clubs

If fitness activities top your checklist of lifetime sports, go to a nearby fitness center, athletic club, or your neighborhood YMCA. Ask if a staff member can give you a tour and explain the equipment, classes, and services offered. If you like what you see and hear, join the facility. If you're not sure it's right for you, ask about a trial or visitor's membership.

In addition to fitness equipment and rooms for aerobics and yoga classes, these facilities may also have courts for racquetball, handball, and squash, or a gym for basketball, volleyball, and other sports. Check it out, and ask if they offer instruction in sports that interest you.

Finally, ask if the facility has personal trainers or other fitness professionals who can serve as your beginning-level coaches.

Educational institutions

High schools, colleges, and universities often offer everything from water polo and fencing to archery and hip-hop dance classes for their students, and may have similar continuing education classes for adults. If a school has courts for badminton, volleyball, handball, racquetball, or squash, it may have instructors to help you learn these sports.

Sporting goods stores

People who work in sporting goods stores are often avid participants in a lifetime sport. Whether it's a specialty shop such as a tennis, golf, or ski store or the paddling, cycling, or camping section in a larger sporting goods store, the staff will likely be active in that sport and know where you can find lessons.

People places

Go on a tour of your town or city and find out where people participate in physical activities. Within a short drive from my home in Santa Barbara, California, population 85,000, are a bowling alley, a riding stable, a golf course, tennis courts, a 50-meter swimming pool, two lawn bowling greens, and a number of dance, martial arts, and yoga studios. These are in addition to several fitness centers, an athletic club, and a YMCA that offers a cornucopia of physical activities. And along the coast

I can find beach volleyball courts, a bike path along the shore, and a skateboard park, as well as sailing and water sports centers that offer lessons and classes. A quick look at the ocean and I can see surfers, ocean kayakers, kiteboarders, windsurfers, and Jet-skiers, as well as a few outrigger teams paddling out past the wharf.

You may be surprised at how many locations for physical activities there are in your hometown—and how many people are having fun exercising at them. Strike up a conversation with someone at one of these locations, and you'll probably learn where to get lessons and find a coach.

Ask the right questions

A word of caution: please sign up only with trained, experienced people or classes that are well known in your community. Once you've identified the locations where you might find a coach and take your first lesson, ask these questions:

➡ *Do you have classes for beginners?*

➡ *Can I get a schedule of classes?*

➡ *How much do the classes cost?*

➡ *When can I check out your facility in person?*

➡ *What are my instructor's credentials?*

Then, ask yourself these questions:

➡ *Is the location convenient—quick and easy to get to?*

➡ *Do the classes comfortably fit my schedule?*

➡ *Are the lessons affordable?*

THE NEXT STEP

With "pleasure is the measure" as your guiding principle, you've checked off activities for your exercise program that are inherently fun to do. This is the first, and perhaps most important step on the road to locking in exercise for a lifetime. By finding a good beginning-level coach to make the learning process enjoyable, you'll learn new skills that will add to your pleasure.

In the next chapter, we'll examine the third way athletes maximize the pleasure of exercise—they share their activity with friends.

Chapter Three

TEAM

The time and effort optimizer

Picture yourself as a competitive swimmer with your eye on Olympic gold. You work out every morning from 6 to 8, and again every afternoon from 3 to 6. Your workouts consist of a series of sets; a typical set might be 20 100-yard swims, with a brief rest between each repeat. Let's face it: if you were working out by yourself everyday, or even with a coach who called out times and encouragement, this would be excruciatingly tedious and boring—and unlikely to maximize results.

> *"At the low end of exertion, you may join a croquet, archery, ping-pong, or lawn bowling club."*

It's one thing to do the swimming; it's quite another to push yourself hard enough to get the results you desire.

Now, if you take that same scenario and add a few more swimmers, you have the makings of an energizing five hours of competition and camaraderie. What might ordinarily be considered hard work—several strenuous hours in the pool—can become a more enjoyable activity when done with others as part of a team.

JEFF JOINS A MASTER'S TEAM *Jeff takes swimming lessons for a couple of years and gradually progresses from a weak swimmer to a lap swimmer to a member of a master's team. Joining a team at age 49 is the step that seals his choice of lifetime sport; he now has a group of friends who share his interest in that sport and challenge him to be the best he can be on a daily basis. Jeff always arrives early to class, joining several teammates for a "warm up" in the Jacuzzi. After a few minutes of motivating camaraderie, he's ready for class and jumps in the pool for the real warm up—a 400-yard swim.*

WHAT WE CAN LEARN FROM ATHLETES

During the 2008 Olympic trials, swimmer Michael Phelps credited his teammates for his success in winning an unprecedented eight Olympic gold medals. Indeed, he said he couldn't have done it without them.[9] Everyday, team members engage in fierce competition, pushing one another to improve. Hard work, yes, but athletes enjoy racing against one another and that makes it fun.

Let's examine how young athletes-in-training benefit from joining a team, and see how to apply those same concepts to your life. There are several factors to consider.

Ease of participation

YOUNG ATHLETES: When kids first try a sport and join a class or team, their motivation is to have fun. The parents may be more pragmatic. They may appreciate that, in addition to teaching their child the skills of an activity, a team makes it easier for them to get their kids involved in that activity in the first place.

Youth team practices generally start right after school, thus parents can build their day around a predictable schedule. Practices take place in fixed locations—soccer players head to the soccer field, ballet dancers to the studio, ice dancers to the rink, bowlers to the lanes, surfers to the beach. The practices provide ongoing instruction; the students can benefit from regular instruction and coaching at every workout. Further, practices provide structure. The coach reserves the location, assembles the team members, provides the equipment, and leads the session. Parents need only pay any fees, drop their children off, and pick them up a few hours later.

Okay, so how does this apply to you?

YOU: Joining a class or team lowers your *response cost*— the total amount of time and effort required to participate in your chosen activity. Initially, your first team will likely be a class where you learn beginning-level skills. Once you pay the class fee, all the logistics are taken care of. Your coach reserves the location, schedules classes, and provides the appropriate equipment. All you have to do is show up.

As you recall, convenience is vital for the parents of young athletes who need to chauffer their kids between activities. Classes and teams provide that same convenience for you, making it easier for you to become a regular participant.

As a rule of thumb, always strive to keep the response cost of your exercise program as low as possible. If participation is easy and convenient, you'll be more likely to continue with that activity.

Fun with people

YOUNG ATHLETES: Kids love to be on teams because sports participation is more enjoyable with friends. On swimming teams, coaches strive to make kids' workouts fun by using sprints and relays along with games like "sharks and minnows." The "minnows" line up on one side of the pool, except for one kid—the "shark"—in the middle. When the coach blows the whistle, everyone tries to swim underwater across the width of the pool. The shark tries to pull minnows to the surface. Gradually the number of sharks grows. The last surviving minnow wins the game and everyone has fun—while they're exercising!

For young athletes, having fun with their friends is a big motivation to stick with a sport.

YOU: The truth is, you'd probably rather be playing sharks and minnows! You'd be bored doing laps by yourself three hours a day. Add another person to your workout though, and it can be a lot more enjoyable. It's human nature to enjoy doing things with other people. Add a pool full of people, and it's a party! For athletes of any age and level, belonging to a group or team can make participation a lot more fun.

When you first join a class, you may not know anyone. As the class proceeds over a period of weeks, however, you'll likely get to know at least one or two new people. You'll look forward to seeing them at class, and they'll connect with you as well. You now have some new friends with whom to enjoy exercise, and your group of friends will increase as you advance to other classes.

If you tend to shy away from groups, you may think you prefer to exercise by yourself. If you've been successful exercising alone, that's great. By all means, continue. But if you've been unsuccessful, try joining a team. It may be the vital difference that can help you stay involved. Keep in mind that you can be relatively independent within a group or class, if you like. You can minimize the level of involvement by arriving just before the session begins, choosing a somewhat isolated position in the group, and leaving immediately after class. Give it a try.

Competition

YOUNG ATHLETES: Parents, coaches, and teachers can motivate athletes to some degree, but nothing breathes life into practice like a little competition. Competition between team members gets kids to focus, try harder, and strive to beat their friends—in a friendly way, of course.

I learned how to compete when I was 12 thanks to a 10-year-old on my first age-group swim team. One day my dad pointed out a 4' 10" swimmer named Dolores and asked me why I couldn't beat her. After all, I was older, close to 6' tall, and (a whopping) 120 pounds. To my chagrin, Dolores was always faster than me. So I developed a strategy: on a set of ten repeats, I strived to beat her on just a couple of them. As I improved and reached my goal, I aimed to win six or seven. Finally, I wanted to win all ten. I was thrilled when I did. As soon as I could regularly beat Dolores, I set my sights on the next fastest swimmer. Through my career, I made a game out of trying to beat the next best swimmer. That game made workouts more fun.

YOU: The desire to win—or simply to do better—may be just the spark you need to succeed with exercise. There are many ways to approach this. You can compete with other class members, just as I did with Dolores. Pick someone slightly more skilled than you, then try to match and exceed that person's skills by the end of the class. The "competition" need not even know about the game! As soon as you've bested that classmate, you can create an ongoing challenge by working your way up the ladder of performers, surpassing one after another.

Imagine taking a spinning class, for instance, riding a stationary bicycle while the instructor periodically varies the pace via the music. When the instructor leads the class into a short up-tempo section, try to keep up with the nearby person slightly better than you. Repeat this over the weeks, and you'll soon be as good, then better than that person—at which point you move on to compete against the next best person in the class.

This concept transfers easily to most any sport, from ice hockey and football to Frisbee, curling, and croquet.

You can also compete against yourself, aiming to master new skills within a certain time. Set a goal to learn a new skill by the end of each class, then push yourself to achieve those skills. If you're learning, say, beginning yoga or country-western dance or stand-up paddling, set a goal to master the basic moves by the end of the class series. If you're a skateboarder or snowboarder, set weekly goals to learn and master new tricks.

Clubs and teams for all abilities

YOUNG ATHLETES: Teams can embrace every level of ability to keep young up-and-coming athletes challenged and engaged—starting with the novice team. As kids improve, they progress to age-group teams and high school teams. If they excel, they may even earn scholarships via college teams. The best of the best then join club teams and compete to earn spots on teams targeting the Olympics and other international championships.

YOU: Adult teams also form around levels of varying ability. You won't find intermediate or advanced students in a beginning class. Once novices acquire the beginning skills of a sport, they can migrate to an intermediate level class and go on to an advanced level class. Whether beginning or advanced, participants tend to have more fun and do best with team members of like ability.

If you were to join an entry-level bike club, it might focus on, say, a recreational Saturday morning ride, with the halfway mark at a restaurant stop for breakfast. One step up in ability, and you'll find bike clubs that place more emphasis on training; members of these clubs are often seen riding in a pack. Finally, there are also clubs that emulate racing teams, training for races of 100 miles or more.

There are clubs and teams for every adult sport and every level of ability. As you progress in skill development, you'll be able to join more advanced teams suited to your new skill level.

SEEK OUT THE POWER OF TEAMS

Your first team: a class

A class usually serves as your first team. Join a class as part of your plan for success, and you'll greatly increase your chances of sticking with exercise for a lifetime. In a class, you participate with a group of people who share your interest in learning a particular activity. In time, some of these people may become your practice partners.

Typically, within six to ten weeks of beginner instruction, you'll be on your way to mastering introductory-level skills—those that allow you to participate in an activity and at least look like you know what you're doing! Once you reach this critical skill level, your instructor may recommend additional opportunities to supplement regular participation.

A note about aerobic classes

If you examine the tremendous success of aerobic exercise classes, you'll see the synergy of coach and team in action. Much like the coach-team experience, an aerobic class transforms repetitive exercise movements into an enjoyable lifetime sport. At a preset time, participants show up for class at a prereserved facility where the equipment is ready for use. They may talk briefly with other "teammates" before the workout begins. The instructor or "coach" has choreographed the workout to music to make it more enjoyable. During the workout, the instructor helps the participants do their best, praises them for their effort, and encourages them to come to the next class.

Over time, participants develop their skills, build up strength and cardiovascular fitness, and progress from beginning- to intermediate- to advanced-level classes.

Clubs or groups

In addition to taking ongoing classes, consider joining a specialty club or group. If you're into dance, martial arts, tai chi, or yoga, you can find studios where people participate regularly in groups. If you're a skier, join a ski club. These clubs often organize trips that include transportation, lodging, and meals. During the summer, that same club—or at least some of its members—may focus on seasonal activities such as cycling, windsurfing, waterskiing, or sailing.

At the low end of exertion, you may join a croquet, archery, ping-pong, or lawn bowling club. No, these are not particularly vigorous activities, but they're much better than not exercising at all. And, as you'll learn in the chapter on supplementary fitness, if you enjoy lawn bowling, croquet, ping-pong, or archery, you might be surprised by your motivation to strengthen your arms, core, and legs to improve your performance.

YMCAs, fitness centers, and athletic clubs also offer recreational activities that may include a tennis, racquetball, squash, or badminton "ladder." These racquet sports ladders offer lots of friendly competition. Participants are ranked according to ability and challenge each other in order to move up the ladder.

For those of you who enjoy hiking, backpacking, rock climbing, river rafting, canoeing, or kayaking, organizations such as the Sierra Club have outings for all ability levels, ranging from regional training hikes to international expeditions. If golf is your passion, visit the public course and ask about clubs for men, women, or couples. It should be easy to find people who share your interest.

LISA BREAKS IN HER HIKING BOOTS *Lisa, 37, loves nature and the outdoors, so she decides to try camping as a lifetime sport. She buys a pair of hiking boots and enrolls in a 20-student beginning-level mountaineering course. During the first two weeks, she learns basic hiking and camping skills. To break in her boots, she takes regular walks through her neighborhood. Eventually she adds a weekly hike to her schedule, exploring the local foothills with a couple of friends from class.*

In week six, the class goes on a weekend camping trip. During the trip, the instructor guides Lisa and her classmates through field activities aimed at mastering their skills, from reading maps and setting up camp to rock climbing and rappelling. The group also enjoys evening cookouts. By the end of the course, Lisa feels comfortable going on camping trips that require hiking into wilderness and making camp.

Meanwhile she begins to build a group of friends interested in active adventures that includes such sports as hiking, river rafting, kayaking, ice climbing, trail running, and zip-lining. She goes on to become an active member of the Sierra Club, pursuing adventure sports with other like-minded athletes and traveling to the far corners of the globe. For Lisa, it all started with a simple class and a willingness to get to know others and share a passion for a lifetime sport.

Teams and leagues

Your local recreation department may sponsor a variety of teams and leagues for adults. Ask how you can join and participate in a bowling, softball, volleyball, basketball, or cricket league. Or perhaps you work for a company that sponsors a team. Ask around.

If you're a swimmer, consider joining a master's team—a swimming team of adults grouped by age—for the regularly scheduled workouts. If you want to enter competitions, you'll vie against others in your age group. For instance, if you're 53 years old, you'll compete in the 50-55 age group; if you're 67, you'll compete against swimmers 65 to 70. Then again, if you're keen on running, consider joining a master's track team that focuses on running and other track and field events. At local or regional competitions, the events are organized so you compete against people of like ability.

While master's teams may include highly skilled individuals, they'll also include people who simply want to improve at the sport and have fun.

Friends and family

Friends can make a wonderful team. A common example is the four friends who play tennis or hike or square dance every weekend. But consider the group of people who meet at an athletic club to play handball on Saturday mornings. They're also an informal team. Friends who go on trips to windsurf, snorkel, snowshoe, or paraglide are a team, too. People who bowl or run marathons together are also a team. The same holds true for friends who enjoy ballroom dancing, scuba diving, sailing, skydiving, riding, mountain biking, water aerobics, or other sports activities as a group.

Families who regularly participate in sports together also function as teams—and can serve as a constant exercise support system for one another. When a family takes up a sport like camping, it can become a favorite activity. Kids can be an irresistible force in motivating parents to go outside and play! If kids enjoy hiking, canoeing, or waterskiing, they'll make sure mom and dad schedule periodic trips to the mountains and lakes. A shared pleasure in mountain or dirt biking can keep a family riding, backpacking, and camping on a regular basis. The same goes for snorkeling, bodysurfing, and boogie boarding at the beach.

The smallest team is the team of two, for example a couple who walk the neighborhood together, play tennis on the weekends, or go out dancing during the week.

Pets

Pet owners and their pets may also function as a team. Start taking your dog for a regularly scheduled walk; you'll soon have an avid walking partner. At the appointed hour, that partner may even stand by the door, waiting for you to pick up the leash and go! Expand your program with runs and hikes. I've enjoyed the help of several furry friends in staying physically active.

Through my 40s, I swam in the ocean and body-surfed with Colby, a black Labrador retriever. My next dog, Juliet, a yellow Lab, loved to play ball and explore the neighborhood with me. Now I have Ben, a 20-pound Tibetan terrier, who always lets me know when it's time for our evening walk. We never miss it. I suspect he's really telling me he wants the doggie treat I give him afterward—but for me, the walk is the treat. In his company, of course.

A word about cost

The cost of lessons and equipment can be a barrier to taking up certain sports. Don't let it be a barrier for you. Every physical activity has some cost associated with it—even walking! If you develop a walking program, for instance, and begin to increase the distance you cover, your shoes will wear out more quickly, and you'll probably want to get a new, more durable pair.

Yet, there are ways to keep your lifetime sport within your budget: joining clubs that provide the equipment, purchasing used equipment, and renting equipment all help minimize the costs of participation.

Sailing might seem the most expensive lifetime sport, given one obviously needs a boat to sail. But if you join a sailing class through your city recreation department, your equipment—the boat—is provided as part of the instruction fee. As your skills advance, you can join a sailing club that rents boats at reduced rates for member use. You can even try learning how to crew on a racing boat. You don't need to own a boat to have lots of fun and get plenty of exercise sailing.

Cycling may also seem an expensive sport. Figure a brand-new, entry-level bike might cost around $400; a midrange bike, $1,500; an advanced road bike, $3,000 or more. Happily, club members moving from $1,500 bikes to $3,000 bikes may offer their old bikes to other members—at near half-price!

Rental equipment from sporting goods stores is another cost-cutting option, and here's another tip: those stores usually update their stock seasonally replacing it with new equipment. Club members often know when those sales take place, and can get their equipment at significant discounts.

One other suggestion: within your budget, try to get the best quality you can afford. Better gear tends to bring greater comfort and ease of use, which enhances the learning experience.

HOW TO APPLY WHAT YOU'VE LEARNED

Here are a few tips for maximizing the benefits of being in a class, belonging to a club, and joining a team.

Be on time
If a class member is five minutes late, the instructor may pause to bring that person up to speed, thereby slowing progress for other class members. And if several people are late, that can delay the start of the class, which allows less time for instruction. This can be especially annoying to other class members who've paid their fee, arrived on time, and are anxious to learn. In the long run, you actually benefit most by arriving a little early

and using those extra minutes to warm up, connect with others in the class, and get to know your instructor.

Smile, smile, smile

When instructors come to class, they have to leave the concerns of the day behind to bring positive energy and enthusiasm to the class. You'll benefit by doing the same. If everyone brings a good attitude to class, everyone has a more enjoyable experience—and, as you know by now, enjoying your exercise program is the key to its success. Even when a day is so hectic you can't leave the stressed feelings behind, you'll soon discover that even ten minutes of moderate-intensity exercise can make those feelings disappear. Exercise is indeed nature's tranquilizer.

Develop friendships

Make friends with two or three people in class, and you'll have two or three new reasons to attend regularly. Miss a session and, at the next session, one of them will surely say, "I missed you at the last class." You and your new friends will unconsciously hold one another accountable for showing up.

If you haven't formed connections with anyone, it's easier to skip a few classes, and it's people without connections to others who ultimately tend to drop out. If you have, say, five good friends in your class, you're much more likely to stick with your routine and succeed with your exercise program.

Some teams may have social activities—another opportunity to get to know your team members and build friendships. Take advantage of these activities. Meeting other participants for coffee before or after class can help you get to know them; the more invested you are in being an active team member, the more likely you'll attend classes regularly.

Help others and allow them to help you

Learning new skills thrives on feedback. If your instructor is working with other students and is unavailable, ask a classmate to observe your skills at practice and provide feedback; you can do the same for them. Building class relationships where you help one another can enhance and expedite your learning.

Share your appreciation

The synergy between coach and team can help you stay involved with exercise for a lifetime. Most instructors put their heart and soul into making their classes enjoyable for their students. A simple "Thanks—great class!" goes a long way in recognizing their efforts.

In the same spirit, if you notice one of your class friends doing something well, mention it to them as you leave. You'll feel good and so will that person. Teams function best when everyone works toward the goal of continuous improvement.

THE NEXT STEP

By creating a routine schedule for your lifetime sport, you can overcome the number one reason people cite for lack of exercise—too little time. In the next chapter, you'll discover how easy it can be to make time for your new sport. We'll examine the strategies that top athletes rely on not only to schedule their sports, but also to maintain a well-balanced life. You'll learn how to use those same techniques to reserve and protect time for your exercise program.

Chapter Four

TIME

The good relationship that begins slowly

The most frequently cited reason for lack of regular exercise is lack of time. Everyone faces a seemingly endless list of commitments that compete for their time, from work and family obligations to social and spiritual activities, community involvement, and leisure pursuits. ▶▶

Between one obligation and another, it may seem like there's little, if any, time left for exercise. Yet people who are successful with regular exercise manage to find that time.

> *"You may start out thrilled with your once-a-week exercise program and decide to do it every day. Resist that temptation."*

When someone says there's no time to exercise, perhaps what they're really saying is, "It's not a priority." Maybe people who are successful at physical activity make exercise a higher priority—maybe they schedule it as regularly as they do eating and sleeping.

Which leads us to the question: Is there an easy way to make exercise a higher priority?

The answer is yes!

WHAT WE CAN LEARN FROM ATHLETES

Tiger Woods's father introduced him to golf at age 2, and the future golf legend loved the game right from the start. Woods learned time management early as well. He memorized his father's phone number at work and called every afternoon like clockwork to ask, "Daddy, can I practice with you today?" In his mind, he had blocked out specific times each day for practice with his father. He started off hitting golf balls every day; over many years that daily visit to the driving range grew into a workout and practice schedule of nearly ten hours per day.[10]

We can learn a lot from the exercise habits of athletes like Tiger Woods. As kids, these future world-class athletes usually started with once-a-week lessons—a minimal time commitment that gradually grew into 20 to 30-plus hours a week.

Children on the path to becoming highly successful athletes go through three stages of development, described by scientists and educators as the "early years," the "middle years," and the "later years." You can approach your exercise program through three similar, scaled-down stages.

I call these the "beginning," "intermediate," and "advanced" phases to correspond with learning beginning, intermediate, and advanced skills.

Developing athletes tend to move effortlessly, almost automatically, from one phase to another. The same can happen to you as, little by little, exercise becomes an exciting new priority in your life.

Know where you're going

You may be wondering at this point how you'll go from a newbie in your chosen sport to someone who has intermediate or advanced skills and has made that sport part of your daily routine. Let's look at how the three stages play out for athletes, and how they can work for you. If you know where you're going and what to expect, you can get there more easily and quickly.

The beginning phase

During the early years, when a future athlete first launches into a sport, the focus is on having fun. The process begins with a minimal time commitment, usually weekly hour-long lessons. At this stage, kids are essentially sampling activities to see which ones they enjoy. If kids enjoy an activity and do well, they might join a novice team, where the focus stays on fun and time commitments remain minimal. If they don't like the activity, they've not invested a lot of time and can move on to something else. If their interest continues, however, they can move on to a more advanced team.

For you, the beginning phase will be the most important one. If you don't succeed with the beginning phase, you'll not want to move on to the next level. In the beginning, think like a 7-year-old, like a young child trying out a new sport: focus solely on having fun. Since you're trying out new activities to see if you enjoy them, keep your time commitments small.

You can start the beginning phase by enrolling in a once-a-week class or a short series of private lessons. One class a week for six to ten weeks, and you'll know whether you like an activity. Much like dating, if there's a spark, you'll want to continue the class. But if three months into it you lose interest, it's time to try something else.

For instance, I once took a Sierra Club beginning-level mountaineering course, ten weekly lessons that covered the basics of hiking, climbing, and camping. While I enjoyed the class, and the skills I learned helped me feel more competent on backpacking trips, I didn't fall in love with mountaineering. (I'm afraid I prefer my camping at a comfy hotel overlooking a golf course.) But one guy in the class was like a mountain goat—learning the skills came easily and naturally for him, and he was clearly having fun as he zoomed up the boulders. I'm sure he went on to become a lifetime rock or mountain climber.

At the beginning level, most teachers, instructors, class leaders, or coaches will recommend a minimal amount of practice, maybe 15 to 30 minutes once or twice a week. In every field of talent—from sports to painting to music—a little practice is essential for improving skills, enhancing performance and enjoying that activity to its fullest.

During this phase, be content to take the lessons and do a little practice. Only when you feel competent in the basic skills is it time to go out and participate.

A golf instructor, for instance, would rarely take a beginning student out on the course until near the end of a lesson series. The reason is simple. The instructor wants the students to have a good first experience on the course. The same holds for learning sports such as squash, badminton, or tennis. At your first tennis class, you may have difficulty just hitting the ball over the net. It seems so easy, but when you get a racket in your hand, the ball doesn't always go where you want. You probably won't be playing any games or sets during beginning lessons. The fun is in learning how to hit a forehand ground stroke, then a backhand ground stroke and other skills such as serving and volleying. Between lessons, your instructor might suggest that you and a partner practice hitting forehands or backhands over the net and try to rally back and forth.

The intermediate phase

The middle years for young athletes are dramatically different from the early years. Coaches who organize sports teams know that kids transitioning to more advanced teams are used to having fun; they also know that those kids need to practice to develop their talent. Therefore, the coaches gradually add increasingly larger doses of practice to the fun. Just as early elementary school has little or no homework, as students progress from elementary to junior high school, high school, and college, the amount and difficulty of their homework increases proportionately.

Talent development requires a gradual increase of time and effort. The coaches of young athletes who went on to become top athletes first increased the frequency of practice days from twice a week to three or four times a week and, later on, to five times a week; along the way, they gradually increased the duration of the workouts from an hour a day to two or three hours and finally, for serious students, to four hours or more.[11]

Your intermediate phase will parallel the development of young athletes, but on a smaller scale. Becoming more skilled in a lifetime sport such as hula or hip-hop dancing, free diving, kiteboarding, jai alai, ice-skating, martial arts, parkour—any physical activity—requires participation more than once a week. Here's the good news: if you really enjoy that activity, you'll find yourself wanting to invest a bit more time in it on your way to the next skill level. You'll be tapping into a natural desire to improve at something you enjoy.

Like athletes with a desire to reach the next phase, you may start by increasing the number of days you participate—maybe from one class a week to two, and from one practice session to two.

Gradually, you may also begin to invest more time each day, increasing from an hour per session to 90 minutes or even two hours.

As a beginner, you're focusing on having fun and performing the basic skills—and sometimes not succeeding with the latter as fast or as well as you might like. You may have yet to actually play a game of cricket or soccer, feel graceful on water skis or snowshoes, or kickbox or roller-skate with ease. All that changes when you reach the intermediate phase. It's during this intermediate phase that physical activities become exponentially more enjoyable.

TED MAKES PROGRESS *In Chapter Two, we followed Ted, the skier who took his first lesson at age 44, as he picked his way down the bunny slope. Having enjoyed that initial experience, Ted* *pursues skiing further. On his next ski weekend, he enrolls in a Saturday morning ski class and, among students of like ability, he improves and refines the basic skills. He also learns new ones. He dedicates his Saturday afternoon and Sunday to having fun practicing what he learned in the morning lesson. He really enjoys skiing and skis six weekends his first season, always reserving Saturday morning for a class. A year later, as an intermediate skier, Ted skis swiftly and confidently down beginning-level slopes and spends most of his time on the intermediate slopes.*

At this vital intermediate stage of development, you can surf—and begin to look graceful on the board. You can rumba and be lithe and agile on the dance floor. If you take bowling lessons, you'll have progressed beyond rolling a straight ball, and can curve the ball toward the pin of your choice. You get the picture. And it's a nice one!

A milestone

Many people are content to stay here at the intermediate level—and why not? Indeed at this point, major congratulations are in order. You've reached one of the most important milestones of success—the intermediate level, where you have the skills to enjoy participating in your lifetime sport.

You're playing regularly, you're having fun—and you're getting regular exercise two to four times a week that contributes to your glowing health and vitality. You've developed a healthy appetite for exercise that can continue for a lifetime. Bravo!

The advanced phase

Of course, some of you may be wondering just how good you might get at your sport if you went further—if you went on to yet the next level of lessons and practiced just a little more.

That's what happens to young athletes who go beyond the middle years. Young athletes who go on to compete at national, international, and Olympic levels tend to put in around 10,000 hours of diligent practice over a ten-year period.[12] Success at this advanced level of competition assumes the athlete has the genetic gifts to be an elite performer.

As an adult who wants to improve your talent, you can do what athletes do, only on an abbreviated scale. For you, the advanced phase is more an extension of the intermediate phase: you'll polish your skills and learn new ones that may bring in the elements of personal style and expression. More significantly, you'll find yourself wanting to increase your time commitment to your sport. Without consciously thinking about it, your lifetime sport will have become a much higher priority in your life.

You'll know you've made significant progress when, somewhere between the intermediate and advanced levels, you start to define yourself in terms of your sport. When people ask what you like to do or if you have hobbies, you'll reply, "I'm a salsa dancer" or "I'm a sailor" or "I'm into yoga" or "I'm an ice-skater."

As we'll discuss further in a subsequent chapter, if you cultivate the idea of making continuous improvement and strive to improve your skills and performance, you'll develop not only a healthy appetite for your new activity but also a burning desire for it.

TIME MANAGEMENT

The best time to exercise

Is there a best time to exercise? Is it in the morning before work, during lunch, right after work, in the evening? Over my career, I've heard this question many times. My answer is always the same: the best time to exercise is when you can be successful at it.

There's an element of personal preference in the choice of an exercise time. If you're a night owl, exercising later in the evening may be the best time for you. If you detest evening as well as morning exercise, your prime time may be late afternoon or early evening, say, right after work. If you're an early bird, exercising at 6 a.m. might be ideal.

I worry a little, though, when I hear an early morning exerciser say, "I like to get it out of the way." Those words suggest that the person doesn't enjoy the activity and is doing it out of responsibility. Or worse—that he or she may have difficulty staying with that activity for a lifetime. As you've learned in previous chapters, it's difficult to stick with something you won't enjoy over the long haul.

Conversely, ask people who rise early to snorkel, do tai chi, or ride their bikes before they go to work, and you may hear the opposite lament: "I wish I had more time for this." This suggests they really love their sport and will probably keep it up long term.

Know your sport's time

Your choice of a lifetime sport may dictate the best times for participation. In other words, when you choose your activity, you also choose the times when you'll participate. If you choose dance as your lifetime sport, classes often take place Monday through Thursday evenings.

In addition, your city recreation department or dance studios may hold dances on Friday or Saturday, often starting around 8 p.m. If you go to clubs with live music, the bands tend to start even later. Figure it's rare to find people line dancing or doing the cha-cha at 7 a.m., so if you choose dance as your lifetime sport, plan on doing it in the evenings.

Compare dance with such outdoor activities as archery, cricket, gardening, rugby, ice-skating, scuba diving, zip-lining, rowing, soccer, ultimate Frisbee, and football. If you choose these activities, expect to spend your daytime having fun with them. For tennis players, days are also favored times to play, and early on weekends in particular. Go to the courts on Saturday or Sunday morning at 7 a.m. and you'll see lots of people.

Scheduling choices are substantially greater if your lifetime sport can take place indoors. Figure you can fence, do yoga and Pilates, body build, practice gymnastics, and play ping-pong or handball just about any day you want, morning to evening. The same goes for activities at health clubs such as stretching classes, Tae Bo, Zumba, swimming in indoor pools, rock climbing on walls, and basketball or badminton on indoor courts.

Traditional fitness activities and classes may be the easiest to schedule into a busy day. Most facilities open around 6 a.m. and stay open until 10 p.m. or later. The equipment is always ready. However, unless you truly enjoy participating in a traditional fitness program, don't let that convenience lead you astray. A fitness program makes great sense for anyone keen to pursue it short-term. But we're trying to develop an exercise program for a lifetime, not just the next few months. Remember: choosing an activity you enjoy is the number one predictor for long-term exercise success.

HOW TO APPLY WHAT YOU'VE LEARNED

Young athletes use basic time management techniques to ensure they have plenty of time for their sports. Let's look at how they do it and then apply that to your own schedule.

Take it slow

Developing an exercise program is like developing any relationship. Start with small steps, build on your successes, and progress slowly. The beginning phase will be the most important for your future success, so let's review the concepts for this phase. For the first three months of your new exercise program, if you commit to just one class a week you can be proud of yourself. If you're having fun, say, taking jazz dance or Pilates or a spinning or riding class once a week, those are all great first steps. Bravo!

If pleasure is your primary motivation, that once-a-week time commitment may soon build to two or three times per week and, later, four or five times per week, much in the same way a person begins dating another person, starting with once a week, then twice a week, then three times a week and so on.

On the other hand, if you're forcing yourself to exercise several times a week but not having fun, willpower may be fueling your new habit rather than enjoyment—and your habit will probably be short-lived.

Good relationships start out slowly, and the voluntary time commitment grows with enjoyment. The same will happen with exercise if you take it slow and have fun.

Block out time for exercise

When young athletes head to college and go through orientation, their coaches might instruct them to draw a one-week calendar on a sheet of paper and fill in blocks of time for their weekly activities. The first priority is to block out time for classes, but equally important to serious athletes is their sports participation. As you might imagine, these athletes base their classes around their sports times!

After these two priorities, comes study time. The remaining hours are for social activities and other aspects of college life. Every day these athletes know exactly what they're going to do and at what time.

For you, creating blocks of time will be easy. In the beginning, you'll be taking an introductory or beginning level class that probably meets just once a week. Therefore, you need to create only a one-hour block of time in your entire weekly schedule. For instance, if you take a beginning-level class every Tuesday from 7 to 8 p.m. for ten weeks, you'll block out that time slot. This will be a regular occurrence for the duration of the ten-session class.

If you enjoy the class and enroll again, you're reinforcing that simple once-a-week schedule. If you take that class week after week, month after month, pretty soon you'll stop thinking about it. When Tuesday arrives, you simply head out to class to have fun. Once that happens automatically, you have created an invaluable habit.

Take any beginning-level class, and you can be sure your instructor, teacher, or coach will recommend practice before the next class session. Once you've had instruction on a specific skill, the quickest and easiest way to master it is practice.

For example, if you take golf lessons, you'll probably learn one or two drills at each lesson. Your instructor will recommend you go to the driving range and practice for 15 to 20 minutes.

If samba dancing is your new lifetime sport, your instructor might suggest 15 minutes of practice one evening in your living room. And if bowling is your lifetime sport, your instructor might suggest you go to the lanes and practice by yourself once a week.

Don't leave practice time to chance

You may be tempted to bypass scheduling practice so you can be spontaneous and keep your options open for other enjoyable activities. You may think you'll just squeeze in a practice session sometime when you're free. That's a recipe for failure. Setting fixed times—etched in granite—will guarantee your long-term success.

PAUL TAKES A MEETING *Paul is good at developing a habit. He loves golf and blocks out a couple hours two days a week to play a few holes right after work. When the clock strikes five, he's out the door. If someone asks if he can stay late at the office to work on a project, he quickly responds, "I'm sorry, I'm heading to a meeting; could I do it tomorrow?" The word "meeting" makes it easy to get to his 5:30 p.m. starting time to "meet" with his golf buddies.*

Don't over-schedule

You may start out thrilled with your new exercise program and decide to block out time for it every day. *Resist that temptation.* The most successful programs seldom develop that way. As we've discussed, most long-term success comes from starting small, experiencing success, and building slowly on that success. That's why I recommend starting with one class per week. If you really like it and want to do more, you can always add a second day later on. If you're going to build an exercise habit to last a lifetime, you'll be more successful if you start with a small habit—one day per week—and gradually build on your success by adding days.

More becomes better

Once you've established a small exercise habit, more is better. If you practice once a week, that's good. Twice is better. Three times a week is better yet. If you continue to enjoy your activity and like making improvements, you'll naturally begin to schedule more and longer practice sessions. But remember: take it slow. Start out with one short session a week until your exercise habit becomes a welcome routine.

Use a scheduling system

Enter your regular exercise times in an appointment book, on your calendar, or in your phone. It's important to schedule time for your beginning lessons in the same place you schedule other daily events. I put my exercise times into my iPhone and then set the alert for two hours before the scheduled time. I also like to write those times in an appointment book at my office.

Protect your exercise times

Ask any school-age athlete to do something during a scheduled team practice and you'll probably get the same answer from all of them: "I can't. I have a workout. Can we get together after practice?" The words "practice" and "workout" carry a lot of weight in their world and allow them to protect their commitment to their sports. You can do the same with yours, using the powerful words "appointment" and "meeting," which resonate in the business world.

If you have a scheduled exercise time right after work and someone asks you to do something that conflicts with that time, simply say, "I can't. I have an appointment." That person will probably respond, almost apologetically, "Maybe we can do it later—or another time?" If you don't think using the word appointment will be sufficient, try the equally powerful reply, "I can't. I have a meeting." Remember, in reality, you *do* have an appointment—with your healthy self! In reality, you *do* have a meeting—between your healthy self, your instructor, and others in your class!

By vigorously guarding your reserved exercise times, you're locking in a habit that will serve you well for years to come.

THE NEXT STEP

Once you find an activity you really enjoy, you'll want to participate more often in order to improve. In the next chapter, we'll discuss how a healthy appetite for your lifetime sport brings new motivation to add a little strength training to your exercise program.

Section Two

Chapter Five

SUPPLEMENTARY FITNESS

Physical fitness as a side dish

In this chapter, we'll explore the possibility of incorporating physical fitness activities into your lifestyle, not as the main focus but in a supporting role.

The American College of Sports Medicine and the American Heart Association guidelines offer two approaches to physical activity.[13] These guidelines include either vigorous-intensity physical activity three days a week, or moderate-intensity physical activity for five days a week.

▶▶

"Instead of health and fitness as your motivation, you'll try fitness training to get better at your lifetime sport."

The guidelines make a clear distinction between moderate activity such as brisk walking, and vigorous activity like jogging or fast walking on a treadmill.

In the research that led to these guidelines, scientists designated physical exertion comparable to brisk walking as the gauge of "moderate-intensity" activity.[14]

On the following page, note that both options include additional strength-training exercises.

OPTION ONE ➡ Do 20 minutes of vigorous-intensity physical activity, three days a week—and eight to ten strength-training exercises of 8 to 12 repetitions each, two days a week.

OPTION TWO ➡ Do 30 minutes of moderate-intensity physical activity, five days a week—and eight to ten strength-training exercises of 8 to 12 repetitions each, two days a week.

JOAN OPTS FOR TRADITIONAL FITNESS *Remember Joan in Chapter One? Joan finds success with Option One—a traditional fitness program. She works with a fitness professional who created an exercise program for her that meets the guidelines of the American College of Sports Medicine and the American Heart Association. Her three-times-a-week program involves 20 minutes of vigorous-intensity exercise on the treadmill, elliptical machine, and stationary bike. For strength, she works out with weights. Joan is happy with her exercise program and sticks with it.*

If you've tried and failed repeatedly with a fitness program similar to Joan's, there's the other approach to consider: Option Two, the alternate route. With this active lifestyle approach, you satisfy the guidelines by participating in one or more lifetime sports to meet the moderate-intensity requirements. You can then supplement your chosen lifetime sport—that's right, your favorite physical activity—with a fitness program in a supporting role.

Olympic swimmer Dara Torres provides a classic illustration for the role of a supplementary fitness program. In 2008 at the age of 41, Torres became the oldest American female athlete to qualify for the U.S. Olympic team—her fifth time to do so. Competing in Beijing, she won the silver medal in the 50-meter freestyle, and two additional silver medals in relays. Her success no doubt hinged on her intensive strength and flexibility program to supplement her pool workouts.[15]

Today's coaches almost universally incorporate physical fitness activities into their training—pro, college, and high school coaches alike. And enthusiasts of all sorts of adult recreational activities use fitness programs to improve their performance.

The supplementary fitness program

Athletes use their desire to develop their talent and improve in their sports to motivate themselves to do strength-training programs. You can do the same: instead of health and fitness as your motivation, you'll try fitness training to get better at your lifetime sport.

When you choose a lifetime sport and strive to develop your talent in that sport, it's highly probable that, at some point along the way, you'll actually have the desire to try strength training to improve your performance.

Look at people you know who are passionate about kiteboarding, dirt biking, river rafting, trail riding, karate, swing dancing, or gardening. They may be taking a supplementary fitness class two or three times a week just to stay in condition for their lifetime sports.

Personalizing your exercise guidelines

You can choose any combination of moderate-intensity activities—comparable in exertion to brisk walking—to meet the recommended minimum guidelines. Say you go for a hike, ride your bike, or do Pilates, yoga, or water aerobics for 30 minutes. Brisk walking on the golf course counts as well (riding a golf cart, however, does not).

While it's true that tennis and golf are stop-and-go activities rather than continuous, the guidelines research tracked total physical activity, including climbing stairs, city blocks walked, and participation in other recreational activities.[16]

BILL AND SUE TAKE A SUNDAY STROLL *Remember Bill and Sue from Chapter One? They found success with Option Two and now swing dance four nights a week at the intermediate level in classes and clubs. Since dance qualifies as a moderate-intensity activity, Bill and Sue practice swing dance daily. Dancing 30 minutes of their 45-minute classes counts as one day toward meeting the ACSM/AHA requirements. To fulfill the five-day requirement, they add a 30-minute Sunday walk.*

If you want more options, go skateboarding, rollerskating, or rollerblading for 30 minutes. Need more to meet the guidelines? How about adding a trail ride, tap dancing, Frisbee golf, a Zumba class, or some dedicated gardening. What counts is the accumulation of exercise, whether from several moderate-intensity physical activities or from just one.

Enhancing performance

If you can get excited about a lifetime sport, you too may develop the urge to supplement that sport with fitness activities. In fact, many of the adults you see at fitness centers are there to improve their performance in a lifetime sport. In the fall, for instance, you'll often find people doing leg presses and leg extensions or taking spinning classes to get their legs in shape for ski season.

Some skiers ride bicycles. For years, I never particularly enjoyed bike riding. That changed when a friend invited me on a ski trip the following winter. I hadn't skied for a couple of seasons and knew my legs were out of shape. So I made a deal with myself: if I could build strength in my legs by winter, I would go on the trip as a reward. Because I love skiing and wanted to do well, I started to ride my bike first for 10 minutes, then 15, then 20 minutes a day. I started out at a leisurely pace, but—caught up in the game of reaching the next level of fitness—I gradually kept increasing the pace and distance. Soon I was riding regularly for longer periods— and enjoying it immensely.

BILL AND SUE ADD TO THEIR PLAN *Bill and Sue continue having fun with swing dance and reach the advanced level of their sport. Knowing they need to be in better physical condition to excel as dancers at this level, they enroll in a twice-a-week weight-training program. Between four days of dancing, one day of walking, and two days of weight training at a fitness center, they now meet the ACSM/AHA minimum guidelines for adequate exercise and—most important—they're still improving* *in their sport and having fun doing it. Bill and Sue's initial reasons to start exercising were to be healthier and look and feel younger. Such goals can help some people succeed with workout-style exercise. But they gained the added motivation to participate in fitness activities because they had fun dancing, became passionate about it, and wanted to improve in their lifetime sport. It's this extra motivation—the desire to improve performance—that pushed them to join a gym and stick with their routine.*

As soon as I reached the goal and completed the trip, I set a goal for the following year, with an even bigger reward: a longer trip as a payoff for getting my legs in really good shape! Driven by the desire to stay in shape for skiing, I've also added weight-training exercises to strengthen my legs even more.

HOW TO APPLY WHAT YOU'VE LEARNED

If you build your exercise program around one or more lifetime sports, the desire to maintain a physical fitness program will eventually occur on its own, just as it does in athletes. But be aware that this desire may take a while to develop.

In the previous chapter, I outlined three stages of an athlete's career and the comparable phases you'll go through in developing your own talent. Fitness training isn't part of the early years, when a young athlete's focus is entirely on learning skills and having fun. In your beginning phase, you too need to focus exclusively on having fun and learning beginning skills; fitness activities don't yet come into play. The desire to add a fitness program occurs in your intermediate and advanced phases.

During a young athlete's middle years, coaches add the element of work and practice to the motivation of having fun by gradually increasing the frequency, duration, and intensity of workouts. It's during this phase that kids begin strength training to improve their performance. Similarly, in your intermediate phase, you'll be mastering your sport's skills and may start to entertain a desire to improve your performance. If you do, it may be time to consider adding fitness activities.

But if you don't yet have that urge, be patient. You'll no doubt experience it in the advanced phase.

In an athlete's advanced phase, a comprehensive fitness program is mandatory if he or she wants to compete at the national, international, Olympic, or professional level. Once you reach your advanced phase, you'll probably want to continue improving and contemplate a physical fitness program to boost your progress. You'll notice that other more advanced participants have a supplementary fitness program and you may want to emulate them to reach the same supercharged levels of success.

Here are the key points: In the beginning, focus all your time, effort, and energy on having fun and learning the skills of your new lifetime sport. Remember, pleasure is the measure. Don't worry for one second about getting sufficient exercise to meet exercise guidelines. By focusing on fun, you'll progress naturally from beginning to intermediate to an advanced skill level. Rest assured that at some point during the intermediate or advanced phases, you'll feel the natural desire to work out as a way to improve your performance. You might find yourself doing a lot more walking, jogging, cycling, or aerobics—and the urge to do so will occur naturally. In the next section, I'll share an easy and innovative technique to help you implement that extra exercise into your new lifestyle.

The Incremental Sneak

Millions of Americans have the desire to exercise. They're motivated to start an exercise program and dutifully set a goal to walk, jog, do an aerobics class, or lift weights four times a week. They meet their three-times-a-week goal the first week, continue to do so for a few weeks or months until they miss one session and then another—until they stop the program altogether.

That vigorous start is what I call the "jump-to-the-goal" strategy; it works for some but fails for many others. I prefer a strategy I call the "Incremental Sneak." I use the term "incremental" because, like many good habits, it starts small and grows steadily with success; "sneak," because you start out quietly with an easy first step and gradually, without big fanfare, sneak up on the final goal.

There's an incremental pace to the development of talent. Coaches know they can't take a child at the novice level (twice a week for an hour) and move him or her straight to the competitive level (four hours per day). Even the most talented child needs to progress gradually, step by step. Children who go on to become world-class athletes tend to start with weekly lessons, then join a novice team that practices, say, twice a week, one hour per workout. Gradually they increase the number of workouts as well as the hours per workout. If at any point along the way the workouts get too intense and the fun diminishes, the kids will quit that sport and move on to something else. For adults learning a new lifetime sport, it's no different.

You ensure your best chances for success by proceeding gradually, in comfortable increments. Let's take walking as an example. To start, limit yourself to two days of walking per week. The idea is to develop a small habit, then build a bigger and stronger habit by gradually increasing the frequency and duration of the activity. Here's the trick: You're going to start with a brisk five-minute walk. That's right, you'll walk just 2.5 minutes in one direction and 2.5 minutes back. It doesn't matter if it's in the morning, during a lunch break, before or after dinner, or in the evening. Just be sure you designate specific days and times that work for you and stick to that schedule. The purpose of this limited schedule is to build the habit of walking at a regular time.

Write your walking schedule in your calendar or appointment book. Or program it into your smartphone so the alarm reminds you one hour before walking and a second alert occurs five minutes before. You'll want to program it as a recurring event; for instance, every Tuesday and Thursday at 5:30 p.m. In the beginning weeks, resist the temptation to do more—but don't allow yourself to do less.

Whether you're tired and stressed, it's raining or snowing, or there's a heat wave of 105 degrees, make sure you always walk for at least five minutes at your scheduled time. When it comes to locking in a habit, the key is to be consistent. See if you can have a string of 20 scheduled days you never miss.

After four weeks, when this tiny habit is taking hold, then—and only then—allow yourself to gradually increase the amount of walking time. For the next month—5 minutes out and 5 minutes back. The following month—10 minutes out and 10 minutes back. Finally—15 minutes out and 15 minutes back for a total of 30 minutes.

After several months, you can increase the frequency of walking from two days to three. If you wish, once that becomes a habit in a month or so, you can increase the walking to four days and then to five days. Your main challenge is to keep your new habit alive. No matter if there's inclement weather or you have a cold, walk at least 2.5 minutes out, then 2.5 minutes back. That will keep the habit going. Remember, you're not limited to 30 minutes, five days a week. You can do 45 minutes or an hour—but don't forget that your ultimate goal is to succeed with exercise for a lifetime. Build a solid habit before you add additional days of walking or increase the amount of time.

Another use for the Incremental Sneak

What if you're entirely out of shape? What if you need to be in better physical condition in order to participate in beginning-level classes in your lifetime sport? The Incremental Sneak may be just the answer—as an ideal way to prepare for your classes. It works like this: with the approval of your doctor, start small and slowly build a habit that can keep you healthy for a lifetime. Five days a week, at scheduled times, start walking:

FIRST MONTH	➡	*2.5 minutes out, 2.5 minutes back*
SECOND MONTH	➡	*5 minutes out, 5 minutes back*
THIRD MONTH	➡	*10 minutes out, 10 minutes back*
FOURTH MONTH	➡	*15 minutes out, 15 minutes back*

At the fourth month, you're walking 30 minutes a day and have reached the guideline minimum recommendation. Well done! Resist the urge to rush this program. If you want to do more, you can increase the duration or the intensity from leisurely walking to brisk walking.

Over time, walking 30 minutes a day will put you in better physical condition, ready to begin lessons in your lifetime sport. Most of the great things in life—achievement, personal success, love—tend to occur incrementally and, once attained, often last for a long time. Resist the temptation to rush the habit-building process. Follow a slow-but-steady strategy for success with exercise and you'll greatly increase your chances for long-term success.

THE NEXT STEP

Whether you use fitness activities as a way to prepare for lessons in a lifetime sport or as a supplement once you've reached the intermediate or advanced stage, remember that slow and easy wins this race. I promise that taking the time needed to ingrain a healthy habit will make all the difference on your way to achieving fitness for the long haul.

Now, are you ready to lock in your gains by taking your healthy new habit to an ever more exciting level? In the next chapter, we'll identify an even more powerful motivator and explore how you can harness it for your lifetime sport.

Chapter Six

CONTINUOUS IMPROVEMENT

A healthy appetite for exercise

How would you like to be so eager for exercise that you could hardly wait to get back to it, day after day? Millions of Americans already feel this way—and you can, too.

You probably know people who surf, snorkel, bike, hike, box, bowl, garden, run, snowboard, ice-skate, bungee jump, or play soccer every chance they get. Bring up their lifetime sports in conversation and they light up, eager to share their experiences. It's clear they have a boundless appetite for their sports.

"Everyone needs feedback in order to improve— even the greatest performers in the world."

What is it about their physical activities that they find so delicious—that has them so enthralled?

A desire to get better

I once asked tennis great Jimmy Connors what keeps athletes motivated. Connors traced a series of circles in the air with his index finger. The circles grew successively larger as they progressed from left to right.

"Getting better," he said.

For this former world champion, as with most every athlete I've ever known, the desire to improve indeed serves as motivator and goal.

SETH AND CODY GO FOR A SKATE PARK *Brothers Seth and Cody love skateboarding and every day after school they practice their sport in their driveway. They have fun working on new tricks, mastering each one before moving on to the next. Riding a skateboard is fun. But if fun were Seth and Cody's only motivation, these teens would be skateboarding all over their neighborhood. Instead, like all motivated athletes, they're keen to improve in their sport. They spend most of their time practicing, setting incremental goals to see just how good they can get. As soon as they master a trick and meet a goal, they immediately set another one. They want to get even better. Eventually, the brothers build themselves a mini skate park—a half pipe and a grind rail—to challenge themselves, practicing even more advanced moves.*

All athletes have the mind-set to make continuous improvement. As soon as they improve, they immediately want to get even better. For athletes, the desire to make continuous improvement is a powerful motivator. When young athletes stop improving, they tend to drop out and try something else; when they keep getting better, they're eager to continue the sport. Athletes who set goals every season and continually improve in their performance will develop a burning desire to achieve excellence in their sports.

Likewise, if you strive to improve continuously, you'll enhance your chances of developing a healthy appetite for exercise that will last a lifetime. Once again, remember that you need to start small. For success with exercise, the process of continuous improvement means setting a small goal, feeling good about reaching that goal, then setting the next small goal.

The link of education

All too often, adults quit taking lessons once they've learned the basic skills of a sport, telling themselves that simply playing more will help them improve. They're right—they will improve—but this is the slowest way to do so.

If you were to go to a golf course with a pro to watch players hit their first drives, that pro could no doubt point out those players who could benefit from lessons and coaching. A nongolfer could do the same. While some people tee off with smooth, rhythmic swings, others look awkward. The difference between the two groups? Education. Awkward players reflect a lack of instruction, coaching, and regular practice. Smooth players tend to combine lessons and practice in order to master a precise and reproducible swing.

If you focus on developing a continuing education program in your sport, you'll improve steadily and increase the pleasure gained not only from the sport but also from a sense of accomplishment. By constantly striving to get better, you increase your chances of becoming passionate about your chosen sport. Which certainly solves the problem of sticking with exercise—

you may even develop an athlete's burning desire for it! When you adopt the athlete's mind-set of always striving to get better, you'll be more likely to take ongoing lessons. You'll be more likely to join a team, club, or class, where you can play and practice with other participants. You may even join a fitness program to improve performance in your lifetime sport.

Let's look at how athletes maximize their opportunities for continuous improvement.

WHAT WE CAN LEARN FROM ATHLETES

Athletes aim to develop their talent, master their skills, continuously improve, and, with luck, become the best at their sport. While their long-term career goals—such as making the Olympic team—set a career direction, their short-term goals are the more powerful motivators. It's the short-term goals that compel athletes to practice diligently, often for a season that might last three to six months. Let's discuss how you can easily apply those same concepts to your own exercise program.

Benchmark success

In the quest to improve, athletes start by setting a short-term goal for the season with something just beyond their reach. For a track runner, this might be a specific time standard for their event. For a rugby, soccer, or softball player, it might be winning key games or reaching a certain rank on the team. At the season's quarter, half, and three-quarter marks, athletes may also set some benchmark goals as intermediate measures of success.

Even if a goal remains unstated, there's some expectation of what will be acceptable improvement—which then becomes the goal. When athletes set a goal they want to achieve, they'll immediately start devising a plan for how to do so. You can be sure that plan will include ongoing instruction, coaching, and plenty of practice.

Here's a tip on goal setting: one measure of a goal's strength is its impact on your day-to-day thinking.[17] If you set a goal and subsequently find yourself constantly thinking about how to achieve it, you have a powerful goal. However, if you set a goal and rarely think about it, let alone how to achieve it, you have a weak goal that will not have much impact on your behavior. If you set a weak goal, you need to go back and revise it so that it stimulates your thinking and guides you into action.

Rely on guidance and feedback

For instruction, aspiring athletes look to their coaches. Among the primary roles of a coach is to teach a sport's skills—beginning skills for novice athletes, intermediate and advanced skills for older athletes. At the beginning of a new season, even top professional athletes start off with a review of the basic skills before moving on to more advanced practice. Indeed, in Jack Nicklaus's instructional classic, *Golf My Way*, the legendary player points to his own career: "Every year, going into a new season, I take a refresher lesson from my lifelong teacher, Jack Grout. We begin at the beginning, with grip and setup, and go right through the fundamentals. There isn't a golfer in the world who wouldn't benefit from a similar periodic checkup."[18]

Coaching also involves observation of, and feedback on, the athlete's performance during practice. The coach then makes comments and advises on corrections. Beginners and pro athletes alike need this feedback. As often as not, they think they're doing one action with their body when they're actually doing something quite different. Take the case with Mark Spitz, who first won seven gold medals in the 1972 Olympic games in Munich. One day, Spitz's coach, James Counsilman, filmed Spitz underwater. After analyzing the footage, Counsilman asked the swimmer to describe his arm movement in the water. Spitz demonstrated his stroke, raising his arm above his head, then pulling it straight down. Counsilman took Spitz into the screening room and showed him otherwise. Rather than pulling straight through, Spitz was actually making a sculling motion—in the shape of an "S"—that shot him into the record books![19]

Here's the vital message: successful athletes from all sports continue to get instruction and coaching throughout their careers. Everyone needs feedback in order to improve—even the greatest performers in the world.

Practice with a purpose

Athletes also do plenty of practice—with the goal of developing precise movements. That old joke about a young man with a violin case asking directions to Carnegie Hall—and the older man responding, "Practice, practice, practice!"—holds true for all sports.

Successful athletes spend more than 90 percent of their time practicing skills and learning how to use them in performance.[20] They may invest two to five hours a day, five days a week, 360 days a year to prepare for just one hour of basketball, a two-minute swimming event, or a 50-second gymnastic routine. The athlete's goal is to learn how to reproduce a precise movement under pressure—whether a fluid golf swing or a crisp turn through the gates of the Giant Slalom.

Likewise, the everyday athlete's goal is also to reliably reproduce a precise movement—perhaps a flawless tai chi posture, a serenely controlled warrior pose in yoga class, or rhythmic outrigger paddling.

In the world of mainstream competitive sports, the most important kind of practice is known as "deliberate practice,"[21] wherein athlete and coach work together, one on one. While the athlete strives to replicate a precise movement, the coach provides feedback on his or her actual movement and advises on how to improve it.

Deliberate practice is an essential tool for learning and mastering new skills. Talent development studies of young athletes have shown that the best predictor of success is the total amount of deliberate practice in their sport during the season.[22] The process often starts with an instructor or coach who assigns drills— repeated movements or tasks that help the student learn a particular skill. The student then practices on his or her own—it's practice with a purpose. At subsequent coaching sessions, the instructor evaluates the student's progress in that skill, gives feedback, and corrects errors.

When the student masters the skill, the teacher challenges him or her with new drills directed at learning the next skill. Students learning lifetime sports from fencing and free diving to horseback riding and belly dancing can make significant progress if they engage in deliberate practice. However, when people reach the intermediate skill level—or as soon as they can enjoy playing the game—they often stop lessons and wind up spending little, if any, time practicing new skills.

Happily, the opposite is also true. If they choose to learn and master new skills in order to see how good they can get—and include a healthy dose of deliberate practice—they'll not only continue to improve, but also continue to enjoy the good feelings that come with developing their talent over a lifetime.

Reap the rewards of achievement

Athletes know that when they reach their goals, they'll rake in the rewards. Some of those rewards are personal, such as the sense of satisfaction that comes with accomplishment or the glow of peer recognition. Other rewards are external: ribbons for kids, medals and trophies for more advanced achievement, and recognition for setting records or attaining All-America or All-Conference status. Another external reward that can motivate young athletes is travel. If they do well, they get to travel to competitions.

As athletes reach higher skill levels, travel expands from regional to national to international competitions— say, a world championship in Rome or the Olympic games in London. Of course, at the pro level there are the obvious financial rewards.

Achieving goals at the end of a season reignites any athlete's passion—he or she wants to improve even more. Before long, that athlete's internal dialog switches from "I did well this season" to "I think I can do even better next season." As soon as a new short-term goal for the next season emerges, the cycle begins once again. I call this "The Getting Better Cycle."

HOW TO APPLY WHAT YOU'VE LEARNED

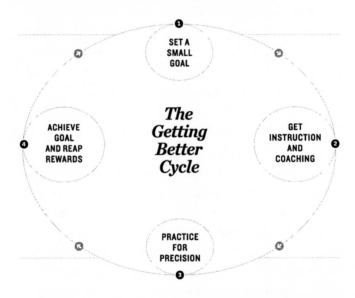

Let's assume you've chosen a physical activity or lifetime sport such as bowling, ballroom dancing, stand-up paddling, or kickboxing, and completed about ten weeks of introductory lessons. You were pleased with the results and have enrolled in the advanced beginning lessons. Now, after 20 weeks, you're able to have fun participating in your activity. After the tango lessons, for instance, you can go to a club and feel competent on the dance floor—you look like you know the basics and can hold your own with your partner and the other dancers. You've reached the intermediate skill level, a significant and exciting milestone in your development.

At this stage you'll face a crucial decision, what I call a "Championship Moment." Do you continue with lessons and practice, or not? When you reach this point, you'll be having fun and may feel content at this skill level. You may choose to stay at that level and believe that frequent participation will help you improve your skills. I urge you to resist this temptation. That's the slower way to improve. Instead, continue taking lessons, keep practicing, and foster a passion for your activity that will keep you interested and excited for years to come.

Here's how to emulate athletes: First, remind yourself that talent development is fun—that continual improvement will add enjoyment and pleasure to your life. Second, put the athlete's mind-set into action by always striving to learn and master new skills. As you improve, strive to get even better. Set your own improvement cycle in motion. You can do it!

Set a short-term goal

ATHLETES: Set a short-term goal for the current season (often spanning three to six months).

YOU: Set a goal to complete a class (often spanning six to ten weeks) or set a goal to learn some new skills.

In physical activities from surfing and rollerblading to ice-skating and yoga, you'll go through the beginning, intermediate, and advanced phases, relative to your ability. Look for a series of classes that parallels this progression. In each class, you'll learn new skills and further refine the ones you already know. Set your short-term goal to complete the next level of class, the one just above your current ability. Think one step at a time. In the pursuit and attainment of each small goal, you'll build a lifetime of fun and satisfaction.

Get instruction and coaching

ATHLETES: Commit to receiving instruction and coaching.
YOU: Commit to receiving instruction and coaching.

Enroll in a class or take private lessons. During the first part of a typical class, the instructor demonstrates new skills and explains the movements you need to learn. This is the instruction portion of the class. You'll then be directed to practice drills on your own, with a partner, or with a small group.

During this segment, the instructor walks from student to student to provide feedback and offer suggestions on how to improve. This is the coaching portion of the class. This combination of instruction and coaching provides the surest and quickest way to learning new skills.

Practice for precision

ATHLETES: Practice 20 to 30 hours per week.
YOU: Practice 15 to 30 minutes, one to three times per week.

Be sure to set aside times to practice the skills you learned in class. If your sport is golf, it means going to the driving range, getting a bucket of balls, and practicing the drills you received from your instructor. If your sport is folk or ballroom or square dancing, you and a

STICK WITH EXERCISE

partner can clear the furniture to create a space to practice the moves you learned in class. For tennis players, it might be rallying with your partner while focusing on one aspect of your forehand volley or cross-court backhand swing. During your practice sessions, remember to focus on performing with precision. This may mean starting out in slow motion in the beginning and, as you improve, picking up the pace. It's learning how to walk before you learn to run!

When I decided to pursue swing dance—a popular activity in my hometown—I wanted to do well in class. To achieve this, I had fun practicing the footwork at home, dancing in slow motion to "In the Mood." By the next lesson, I felt comfortable with the basic steps; at subsequent dance classes I was pleased that I could do the steps at regular dance tempo. That felt great and I stuck with my lessons.

Achieve goal, reap rewards, repeat cycle

ATHLETES: Achieve a goal and get medals, trophies, and other forms of recognition. Repeat cycle.

YOU: Attain the next skill level and enjoy the rewards. Repeat cycle.

At the end of a class series, you'll have learned the skills and will feel personal satisfaction—a sense of accomplishment—about your success. You set a goal to complete a class. You received instruction and coaching. You practiced diligently, finished the series, and reaped the rewards. If you worked hard in class and at practice, you may experience the peer recognition that comes with doing well in a group. These are the internal rewards.

You can also create external rewards that will help motivate you to continue your lessons and practice. For instance, after you complete a beginning-level stand-up paddling class, get yourself a new wetsuit. After you complete the beginning series of lessons in Latin dance, reward yourself with new dance music for your practices or a sizzling new tango outfit.

Consider going a few steps further by creating more external rewards. Adding external rewards can amp up the power of a goal to get you thinking about achieving it, and guide your actions. After completing, say, the first three months of lessons, reward yourself with dinner at your favorite special-occasion restaurant. After six months of lessons and practice, how about an afternoon of revitalizing at your neighborhood salon or day spa? After a year of success, reward yourself with a getaway to one of your dream destinations where you can indulge 24/7 in your newfound passion—your favorite sport!

Above all, each milestone marks a time to restart the cycle, just as athletes set a new goal for the next season.

Assuming you enjoyed the classes, you'll soon be looking ahead toward learning more advanced skills. You'll be ready to set your next goal, completing the next class to reach the next skill level. If you commit to this goal-setting cycle as an essential part of your lifetime sport, you'll continually raise the enjoyment factor while improving your performance. You've come full circle: before you know it, you'll discover a passion not only for your sport but also for the pursuit of continuous improvement.

THE NEXT STEP

We've examined how ongoing lessons and practice are the quickest ways to improve and the surest ways to achieve long-term success with exercise. Yet most of us will be tempted to skip this advice, forsaking lessons and practice for more frequent participation as a strategy to improve. How do we resist this urge? The next chapter will show you how to "just do it"—to stay on track, keep practicing, and enroll in your next series of lessons. Learning these skills may be the most important lesson for achieving your goal to succeed with your lifetime sport.

Chapter Seven

CHAMPIONSHIP MOMENTS

How exactly does one "Just do it"?

Some of my favorite commercials are the Nike spots that show athletes in training, sweating and exerting substantial effort to improve their performances.[23] At the end, you see the Nike logo and the words "Just do it." It's an inspiring sales pitch, but it may leave you wondering, "How exactly do I get myself to 'just do it'—especially when I don't feel like doing it at all?" Figure that out, and you're on your way to a new relationship with health and fitness.

▶▶

"I can promise you that mental toughness is not a God-given trait."

Each year, tens of millions of people set a New Year's goal to exercise regularly. For most of them, it involves a resolution to go to a fitness center several times a week. Some keep it up for a month, maybe two. But then comes that moment of decision: whether to skip exercise—just this once. If they skip exercise once, it becomes that much easier to skip the next session. Each skipped session makes it easier for people to decide to skip it yet again until they rarely work out at all. Or stop. At least they're not alone—70 percent of Americans lack adequate exercise. Which brings to mind all those well-intended American attempts at dieting.

Let's say Carla sets a goal to lose 20 pounds. With the guidance of a dietitian, she develops a sustainable, realistic eating plan. Over the course of a year, she loses the weight and then stays slim for the rest of her life. "Just do it"—right? It's a wonderful vision, but unfortunately one that seldom occurs. Somewhere along the way, Carla will be tempted to improvise or deviate from her plan. She'll give in to temptation. The second deviation will be easier than the first, and each subsequent deviation will be easier still. Soon she's back to her old habits. The lost weight returns. Sound familiar? It's this same scenario that repeats itself with exercise programs.

If people had the power to control their decisions at that moment of temptation—when inertia seeks to highjack action—they'd easily stick with their diet and exercise plans. I call these junctures—when you can choose to prevail over a self-defeating impulse—Championship Moments, a term I came up with while training college athletes. College athletes frequently face temptations to miss practices or loaf a little during workouts when they get fatigued. But they quickly learn that making self-defeating decisions leads to lower performance in the long run. Just as quickly, they learn that making good decisions leads to championships.

Furthermore, if strategies for controlling decisions were available to everyone in their Championship Moments, then tens of millions of Americans would be fitter and healthier (and no doubt slimmer as well, but that's another story). The truth is, these strategies do exist. Not only do you have the power to control your decisions but there are also easy techniques you can learn to strengthen your ability to do just that.

Here's the key concept: the Championship Moment is that space in time when you decide whether to stick with your plan or not. If you make good decisions at your Championship Moments, you progress toward your goal; if you make poor decisions, you fail to reach your goal or you progress more slowly. Your ability to control your thinking at these junctures will determine your success. By simply recognizing your Championship Moments and controlling your decisions, you'll make progress toward your goal and feel good about yourself.

WHAT WE CAN LEARN FROM ATHLETES

If you watched the 2008 Summer Olympics, you saw swimmer Michael Phelps win those unprecedented eight gold medals in Beijing. You also saw him win the 100-meter butterfly by one one-hundredth of a second. Had he skipped just a few workouts, or loafed during practice, he might have placed a respectable second—and missed his chance to rank as one of the greatest athletes in Olympic history!

Like the rest of us, athletes face Championship Moments all the time. This is especially true in a sport like swimming, where one-tenth of a second can make the difference between first and third place. When I look back on my college career as a swimmer, I'm painfully aware of opportunities missed because I made poor decisions and deviated from my plan. As a result, I lost a second NCAA title by one-tenth of a second. If I'd only known then what I know now!

Back then, it would have helped if I'd understood the concept of Championship Moments and knew how to recognize them—and if I'd had strategies for making good decisions at those key moments. While I did well, I could have done better. On the other hand, my greatest successes were preceded by consistently good decisions at Championship Moments. The season I won an NCAA swimming title for the 200 individual medley, I stuck with my plan.

MARK FACES A CHOICE *Mark, 22, a senior in college, is a top athlete on the men's swim team. At the beginning of the season, he sets a goal to win an NCAA championship. He works with his coach to develop an exercise plan that includes daily morning and afternoon workouts plus supplementary weight training three days a week. One chilly morning, Mark's alarm goes off at 5:30 a.m. He wakes up groggy and tired. The night before he studied late. He faces a 15-minute walk to the pool. Mark wants to sleep in. He begins to rationalize how missing just one workout won't hurt his chances of winning. He has come to a Championship Moment. If Mark sleeps in, he may be on the road to his greatest failure, perhaps swimming just a tenth of a second slower than other swimmers and falling short of his goal. If he gets up and goes to practice, he'll continue on the road to winning the championship. With luck and hard work, he'll look back and recognize that his gold medal arose from good decisions at everyday moments like these.*

The most successful athletes rely on mental strategies to help them make the right decisions. You can do the same. With a few simple techniques, you too can consistently make good decisions aimed at doing your best.

The choice is yours

Imagine you're at your own Championship Moment. Let's say you're driving to your exercise class after a tough day, wrestling with two internal voices locked in an argument. One of them is your defeatist self. This is the voice making the case for skipping exercise "just this one time."

Of course, the defeatist self aims for a life of ease and inertia to avoid goal-setting, hard work, or self-discipline.

The defeatist self specializes in denial of its negative affect on your well-being. If you're debating whether to go to the gym or head home after work, the defeatist self says:

➡ It won't matter much if you skip exercise this one time.
➡ You've had a hard day at work. You deserve a break.
➡ Wouldn't you rather relax with a glass of wine and your favorite news show, or spend extra time with the kids?

The other voice, your healthy self, wants you to be the best you can be—active, energized, and looking and feeling great. It encourages you to set goals, work hard, reap the rewards, and stick with your plan. It says things like:

- ➔ You can do it. Just drive to the workout.
- ➔ You'll feel good once you get there.
- ➔ Remember how you enjoy it once you start moving?

This internal dialog occurs naturally whenever you debate an important decision. The defeatist self will start its sabotage, going on about why and how you might get away with deviating from your plan. But if the healthy self gets those last few minutes leading up to the Championship Moment, you'll be more likely to make the right choice. The goal is to manage your internal dialog as you make the final decision.

HOW TO APPLY WHAT YOU'VE LEARNED

Since Championship Moments occur in the mind, the solution lies in the mind as well. Let's look at four key techniques that athletes use—the psyche-up, the self-con (my personal favorite), mental toughness, and visualization—that can help you strengthen your resolve at your Championship Moments.

The psych-up

Focusing on your goals and rewards increases your chances of making a good decision at the Championship Moment—it helps you psych up for class. Begin by focusing on your goals and the rewards.

In effect, you have a talk with your healthy self, who says: "Good for you for committing to physical activity for a lifetime. Do you really want to achieve that goal or not? Once you get to class, it's always fun. Your friends will be happy to see you when you walk in. And remember, you've promised yourself that weekend getaway if you finish all ten classes. Are you really going to let that go? It's time to take action. Let's get moving."

This strategy becomes even more powerful if you start focusing on goals and rewards before it's time to go to your class rather than when you're en route. That way—if and when the Championship Moment arrives—you'll have heard a steady stream of reasons and benefits for making a good decision and sticking with your exercise plan.

The psych-up has an added bonus. When you listen to your healthy self and make a good decision, not only will you stick with your exercise plan but also your self-esteem rises—you'll feel good about your actions. In turn, you'll have more energy to make a healthy choice the next time. Like all the mental strategies, this creates a self-rewarding cycle: when you make a good decision, you feel good about yourself, your self-esteem rises, and you have more energy to stick with your plan.

MARK GIVES HIMSELF A PEP TALK *As Mark rolls over in bed, he's already thinking how good it will feel to sleep in and how missing one workout won't matter. He purposefully interrupts that line of thinking and directs his focus toward his goal and the rewards that may lie ahead.*

"Do I really want to win this event?"

"How would it feel to climb to the top of the awards stand?"

"Do I want that medal and the good feelings that come with winning? I'll be graduating soon, so this is my last chance." By

consciously directing his thoughts to the goal, he effectively
controls his internal dialog. He climbs out of bed, dresses
quickly, and is on his way to the workout. Now he's recommit-
ted and excited about his goal—psyched up.

The self-con

If focusing on the goal didn't work as well as you'd like, and the stoplight is just about to change, it may be time for a self-con. Self-cons are about overcoming inertia and building momentum. Each con moves you one step forward in your plan.

To start, think to yourself, "I'll just drive to the class and park outside. If I still feel tired, I'll start the car again and drive home." As you have these thoughts, make the turn and drive to the class. This first self-con gets you to the class, and in most cases that's enough.

If not, and you're still feeling tired, maybe you need an additional con.

Try this one: "I'll just pop in and say hello to a few people. If I'm still tired, I'll tell them I just stopped by to say hi or to pick up my gear on the way to a meeting." By now, you've paid the lion's share of the response cost—the time and energy to get to class—and you'll probably stay.

However, if you're still feeling tired, you have one final con: "I'll just suit up and start class. If I'm not feeling into it after five minutes, I'll slip out and head home." By this time, the dual powers of exercise as a natural stress reliever and energizer will be taking hold, and odds are in your favor that you'll enjoy your class.

MARKS BACKS INTO HIS GOAL *When Mark arrives at the pool, he looks at the workout board. The sets his coach has listed for him include 20 100-yard swims or "repeats," with only about 15 seconds of rest between each one. Mark knows the first ten repeats will be relatively easy, the next five somewhat tougher, and the last five grueling. When he starts to wear out, Mark could trying psyching himself up to reach his goal. Instead, he goes for the self-con. After number 16, he thinks, "I'll push for just one more and then ease up." When he completes number 17, the con continues: "I'll do one more repeat and then I'll ease up." After number 18, he revisits the con: "I don't have much left. I might as well use it all on this one. At least I will have done a good job on 19 of the 20 swims." Of course, on the last repeat, he thinks, "I have only one more to do, then I can loaf the next set." In the end, Mark succeeds in pushing himself hard his entire set. Is he exhausted? Yes. Is he feeling good about himself? Definitely.*

Mental toughness

For athletes, the psyche-up or self-con are often enough. But what if they both fail? Then athletes rely on a third strategy—mental toughness.

If you ask anyone competing against swimmer Michael Phelps or tennis champ Serena Williams to describe what makes those particular athletes so great, you'll often hear the words "mental toughness." I can promise you that mental toughness is not a God-given trait. It's taught by parents, emphasized by teachers, and reinforced by coaches. Studies have shown that the parents of top athletes place a great deal of emphasis on working hard, doing one's best, and striving for achievement. The parents often model a strong work ethic themselves and expect their children to uphold the same values. These lessons don't stop at home. The message is repeated in schools, where teachers emphasize that doing homework and studying hard leads to better grades, underscoring the relationship between hard work, discipline, and achievement.[24]

Finally, coaches encourage athletes to set goals—and reinforce the message that hard work and self-discipline lead to achieving those goals. Implementing these learned principles over a period of years toughens young kids into seasoned athletes who can simply take control of their actions.

Like budding athletes, most of us heard about responsibility, hard work, and self-discipline from our parents, teachers, and coaches. Would you have more self-discipline if you still had someone you trusted to frequently and gently remind you about the value of exercise?

If so, why not entrust yourself to be the gentle deliverer of those reminders? Try purposefully thinking about the rewards of hard work and self-discipline as a way to simulate gentle parental reminders. Then, when Championship Moments pop up, challenge yourself by asking the questions:

➺ **Am I taking responsibility for my exercise program?**
➺ **Am I being self-disciplined by going home?**
➺ **Am I willing to go the distance to achieve the goal?**

MARK COACHES HIMSELF *From an early age, Mark got the message from his coaches: hard work leads to attaining goals. If he was tired and wanted to ease up during his pool workouts, those coaches cut him no slack. Instead, they urged him to toughen up and work even harder. Now on the verge of winning an NCAA title, Mark relies as much or more on himself as he does on his coach for those reminders to toughen up—and stick to the goal at hand.*

In some cases, taking 30 seconds to answer these simple questions may be sufficient to get you to make the turn toward class. You don't need the mental toughness of an Olympic athlete or a drill sergeant. You don't need to be mentally tough all the time. You just need to be mentally tough for 30 seconds at a time, right before the Championship Moment.

Visualization

Athletes excited about reaching a goal invest a good deal of time thinking about it. They picture themselves in performance, often in great detail. Whether they call it daydreaming or visualization, it serves them well as valuable rehearsal for an upcoming event. It also keeps the goal fresh in their minds.

You're no doubt familiar with the self-improvement philosophy of "you are what you think," which asserts that positive thoughts encourage positive outcomes while negative thoughts yield the opposite results. Whether you believe it or not, thinking in great detail about your exercise program in positive terms can be a valuable tool—a mental rehearsal to help keep you on track. You might picture yourself driving to class, reaching the stoplight at the intersection, and being tempted to skip exercise.

Now the rehearsal begins. You think through your goals and rewards as a way of psyching up. You imagine the self-con and making the right decision. You might even hear yourself asking questions about responsibility and self-discipline.

MARK PICTURES A WIN ➡ *Mark has several opportunities during the day when he can think about winning the championship. While strolling across the campus from one class to another, his mind is in another space. He's thinking in-depth about his upcoming event. Numerous times during the day, he pictures himself diving into the pool, swimming two lengths of butterfly, and having a small lead. Then he visualizes swimming two lengths of backstroke and breaststroke, opening up a big lead. He sees himself swimming freestyle, doing a flip turn at the wall, finishing strong to win the event.*

Now picture yourself making the turn toward exercise: You're performing well. You're learning new skills. You're feeling the sense of pride and accomplishment that arises from following through on a healthy choice. Add to your visualization the good feelings of self-esteem that come when you win at your Championship Moments. Later, when you reach a real-life Championship Moment, you'll be ready to quickly and easily make the decision you've already rehearsed in your mind.

Give your healthy self the edge

At your Championship Moments, it's time to refocus your thinking with the psyche-up, the self-con, mental toughness, or visualization to give your healthy self the advantage. Equipped with these four simple techniques, you can strengthen your resolve just as top athletes do— and succeed at exercise for a lifetime.

THE NEXT STEP

You're making a real and lasting change in your life to "just do it," whether by psyching yourself up, doing the self-con, summoning 30 seconds of mental toughness, or picturing yourself successfully engaged in exercise. You've got the tools. In the final section of this book, you'll find a summary guide to help you set your first few goals and plan your course of action. Human nature being what it is, you'll soon face a choice to follow the best practices outlined in this book or not—your first Championship Moment. Listen to your healthy self, move forward, and discover the wonders that commitment to that plan can hold for you. Be bold and see what happens.

Back in 1951, mountain climber and author W. H. Murray noted a curious phenomenon that kicks in the moment you commit to an endeavor. He said all sorts of elements come into play to help you in your quest that would never happen otherwise—unforeseen incidents and meetings and material assistance that no one could ever dream would come to pass.[25]

"Whatever you can do," he said, "or dream you can, begin it. Boldness has genius, power, and magic in it. Begin it now."

With a fresh new perspective on the best practices for exercise success, and boldness in your spirit to "just do it," it's time to embark on a lifetime of success with exercise.

Are you ready? The answer is yes!

Chapter Eight

SUMMARY & QUICK REFERENCE
Ready, set, go—a course of action

Congratulations on finishing the previous seven chapters of this book. You now know the best practices for exercise success. You also know that millions of everyday athletes use the same set of best practices to stick with their lifetime sports. The diagram below represents these best practices at work. Keep this book handy as a guide for your exercise program. You may want to revisit certain sections, and you can refer to this chapter as a quick reference whenever you need to review an idea or concept. Early success at each stage of the cycle will help ensure your success at subsequent ones.

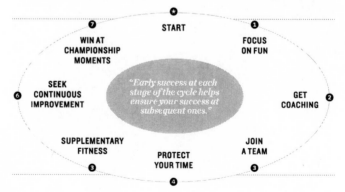

Chapter I | FUN

Having fun—truly enjoying a physical activity—is the key to long-term success with exercise. Most world-class athletes learn their sport as children, when their primary motivation is to have fun. Only later, after they start to excel, do their parents invest time and effort in training. The single most important step you can take toward succeeding with exercise is to choose a physical activity you believe would be fun to do for a lifetime.

ACTION: Your first step is to identify one or more physical activities you think would be fun to enjoy over a lifetime. The guidepost for choosing an activity? Pleasure is the measure!

BENEFIT: When it comes to exercise, it's easiest to stick with physical activities you find fun, enjoyable, and satisfying. Health and fitness arise automatically as a side benefit of enjoying your preferred activity—your lifetime sport.

Chapter 2 | COACH

All athletes benefit from the guidance and encouragement of their coaches. Once you've chosen a lifetime sport, find a coach—a beginning-level instructor who can teach you the basic skills of that sport and encourage you to practice—and enroll in a class or private lesson. Doing so greatly increases your ability to succeed with exercise over a lifetime.

ACTION: Find a "coach"—also known as teacher, trainer, instructor, or class leader—who can help you enjoy your initial experience in your lifetime sport, foster early success in that sport, and set you on a lifetime course of continuous improvement. Then enroll in your first lesson, class, or lesson series.

BENEFIT: Having a coach you trust, respect, and like virtually guarantees success at learning a new activity, and can guide your talent development for a lifetime.

Chapter 3 | TEAM

For young athletes, having fun with friends is a primary motivation for trying a new sport and sticking with it. Athletes belong to a variety of teams during the course of their career, and reach top levels of achievement with the help of team support. A team brings together a group of people who share an appetite for a particular sport. For many people, a shared activity is more enjoyable than doing that activity alone.

ACTION: Team up with one or more people (even a furry friend!) who share an active interest in your lifetime sport. Join a class, club, or league to enhance your chances of success.

BENEFIT: Membership on a team generally provides not only fellow participants for camaraderie and encouragement, but also regularly scheduled times and locations for participation. In addition, it can reduce the response cost—the total time, effort, and expense—required to participate in that sport.

Chapter 4 | TIME
Athletes have fixed times for play, for participation in their sport. They also have fixed times for practice, for improving and mastering skills. These times should be scheduled religiously—and etched in granite.

ACTION: Develop fixed times for lessons, practice, and participation. Use the words "appointment" and "meeting" to protect those times.

BENEFIT: Regular participation in a lifetime sport is essential for success—as is practicing the skills of that sport. Both are sources of fun, enjoyment, and satisfaction. Having fixed times for play and practice will help establish the role of exercise in your life and ensure its priority.

SECTION II

Chapter 5 | SUPPLEMENTARY FITNESS
Athletes do supplementary strength-training activities to improve their performance. As you develop your talent in your lifetime sport, you'll have a desire to improve your performance as well. This is the time to develop a supplementary fitness program of your own.

ACTION: Don't introduce a supplementary fitness program too soon. Your first goal is to establish a habit of regular participation in your chosen lifetime sport. Once that habit is comfortably in place, you'll find you want to improve in your sport. That's when should you add a supplementary fitness program to your schedule. If you're extremely out of shape, you may want to try a walking program and a minimal strength-training program to achieve a sufficient level of fitness to start your lifetime sport.

BENEFIT: Improvement in your lifetime sport through a supplementary fitness program means added motivation to stick with that sport—and succeed with exercise!

Chapter 6 | CONTINUOUS IMPROVEMENT

All athletes set short-term goals for making continuous improvement in their sport.

They get regular instruction and coaching, and devote considerable time to practicing skills in order to reach each goal.

Achieving that goal feels good, which compels them to immediately set a new goal.

ACTION: Emulate athletes by setting small goals for improvement. Take lessons, get coaching, and practice until you reach your goal and gain the rewards of your accomplishment. Soon you'll want to set a new goal.

BENEFIT: Goal-setting can help you improve continuously and retain your interest in your sport for a lifetime. By rewarding yourself for achieving your goals, you'll add to your enjoyment of that sport.

Chapter 7 | CHAMPIONSHIP MOMENTS

Athletes use mental techniques that help them stick with their plans for success. Techniques for prevailing at those Championship Moments—at challenges to their plans—include the psyche-up, the self-con, mental toughness, and visualization.

ACTION: When you're tempted to deviate from your exercise plan, use these techniques to guide you past self-sabotage. Get yourself to "just do it": psyche yourself up by focusing on your goals, plans, and rewards. Con yourself into taking the next small step. Use mental toughness to drive yourself forward. Or visualize how you'll win.

BENEFIT: With practice, you'll become adept at these techniques and well equipped to succeed with exercise.

Chapter 8 | SUMMARY

Here are my biggest hopes: You'll choose a fun lifetime sport, take a class or get individual instruction, and have a wonderful initial experience. You'll pursue that sport through coaching and lessons by joining a club, team, or group that supports your efforts. As a result of those lessons and coaching, you'll enjoy early and ongoing success in your sport. As your desire for continuous improvement grows, you'll discover a new motivation to do supplementary fitness activities. And in using this best practices approach, you'll develop a mind-set for exercise success that will carry you for a lifetime.

That's it—have fun and "just do it." Remember, pleasure is the measure. You're on your way!

ENDNOTES

1 Charlotte A. Schoenborn, Patricia F. Adams, *Health Behaviors of Adults: United States 2005-2007*, National Center for Health Statistics, Series 10, No. 245, Centers for Disease Control and Prevention, (U.S. Department of Health and Human Services, March 2010).

2 Kenneth H. Cooper, *Aerobics*, (M. Evans, 1968).

3 Benjamin S. Bloom, *Developing Talent in Young People*, (Ballentine Books, 1985).

4 Tim Gibbons, et al, "Reflections on Success," *Olympian Report*, (United States Olympic Committee, 2003).

5 "Lindsey Vonn: More About the Athlete," Olympic Medalists, (olympics.org).

6 Benjamin S. Bloom, *Developing Talent in Young People*, (Ballentine Books, 1985).

7 Ibid.

8 Ibid.

9 Kevin Van Valkenburg, "Phelps Completes Historic Quest," (*Baltimore Sun*, August 17, 2008).

10 Earl Woods, *Training a Tiger*, (HarperCollins, 1997).

11 Benjamin S. Bloom, *Developing Talent in Young People*, (Ballentine Books, 1985).

12 William G. Chase, Herbert A. Simon, "Skill in Chess," (*American Scientist: 61*, 1973). K. Anders Ericson, et al, "The Role of Deliberate Practice in the Acquisition of Expert Performance," (*Psychology Review*, July 1993).

13 William L. Haskell, et al; *Physical Activity and Public Health*, (American College of Sports Medicine and the American Heart Association, 2008).

14 Ibid.

15 Elizabeth Weil, "A Swimmer of a Certain Age," (*New York Times Magazine*, June 29, 2008).

16 William L. Haskell, et al; *Physical Activity and Public Health*, (American College of Sports Medicine and the American Heart Association, 2008.

17 Edwin A. Locke, et al, *A Theory of Goal-Setting & Task Performance*, (Prentice Hall, 1990).

18 Jack Nicklaus, *Golf My Way*, (Simon & Schuster, 2005).

19 James E. Counsilman, *The Complete Book of Swimming*, (Macmillan, 1979).

20 Jim Loehr and Tony Schwartz, *The Power of Full Engagement*, (Free Press, 2004).

21 K. Anders Ericsson, *The Road to Excellence*, (Psychology Press, 1996).

22 Ibid.

23 Nike's "Just Do It" advertising campaign (Wieden+Kennedy, 1988).

24 James E. Loehr, *The New Toughness in Training for Sports*, (Plume, 1995).

25 W. H. Murray, *The Scottish Himalayan Expedition*, (J.M. Dent & Sons, 1951).

ACKNOWLEDGEMENTS

I wish to thank the many people who have contributed to this book. In particular, I am grateful to Bob Bartels, my coach at The Ohio State University, for helping me reach my potential as a swimmer and inspiring me to a career in exercise physiology; to Brian Murphy at Occidental College, who showed me how to motivate athletes to do their best; and to all the students and athletes who made my own coaching efforts over the years worthwhile. In addition, I am indebted to my editors: Trish Reynales provided invaluable guidance in seeing the book through from concept to completion; Annette Burden encouraged me to write and helped me get the project off the ground; Linda Jones lent her fine eye for detail. Thanks also to my respected colleagues Eric Durak, Dan Halvorsen, Gary Scherer, and Alan Hedman, who expanded my focus from athletic performance to health and wellness, and provided many thought-provoking conversations along the way. And to my friends Everett Stevens, Don Donaldson, and Diana Lewallen for their cameraderie and enthusiasm. Finally, I would like to thank my parents, classic "everyday athletes," who gave me tremendous support in all my endeavors, and my wife, Debra, for her brilliant insights and unflagging passion for this book.

ABOUT THE AUTHOR

Robert Hopper has assisted thousands of adults in realizing their fitness goals. The author and wellness speaker's previous books include the bestselling textbook *The HSA Strategy* (2006) and *Healthcare Happily Ever After* (2007). Hopper attended The Ohio State University, where he won an NCAA swimming championship and set the American record for the 200 individual medley in 1965. Hopper earned his PhD in exercise physiology in 1977 at the University of Southern California. At Occidental College, he taught the health benefits of exercise and served as head coach of the men's swimming and water polo teams. He went on to found a health-management company, creating corporate wellness programs, followed by a private insurance agency. In 2007, Hopper was honored with membership in the Occidental College Aquatics Hall of Fame. In 2009, he was inducted into The Ohio State University Varsity "O" Hall of Fame, joining the ranks of such athletic stars as Jesse Owens and Jack Nicklaus. He lives with his wife in Santa Barbara, California. His lifetime sports include golf, cycling, and skiing.

CPSIA information can be obtained at www.ICGtesting.com
Printed in the USA
LVOW052044050613

337140LV00001B/95/P